RYPINS' INTENSIVE REVIEWS

Community

Health

Richard H. Grimm, Jr., M.D., M.P.H, Ph.D.

Rueben Berman Professor of Clinical Epidemiology
Director, Berman Center for Outcomes and Clinical Research
Hennepin County Medical Center-Minneapolis
Professor of Medicine and Epidemiology
University of Minnesota

LIPPINCOTT WILLIAMS & WILKINS
A **Wolters Kluwer** Company

Philadelphia · Baltimore · New York · London
Buenos Aires · Hong Kong · Sydney · Tokyo

Acquisitions Editor: Elizabeth A. Nieginski
Editorial Director of Development: Julie P. Scardiglia
Senior Managing Editor: Amy G. Dinkel
Marketing Manager: Christine Kushner

9 8 7 6 5 4 3 2 1

Library of Congress Cataloging-in-Publication Data.

Grimm, Richard H.
     Community health / Richard H. Grimm, Jr.
        p. ; cm. — (Rypins' intensive reviews)
     Includes index.
     ISBN 0-397-51558-8
     1. Public health—United States.   I. Title.   II. Series
     [DNLM: 1. Community Medicine.   2. Community Medicine—Examination
Questions.
W 84.5 G864c 2000]
RA445 .G75 2000
362.1'0973—dc21   99-054062

Care has been taken to confirm the accuracy of the information presented and to describe generally accepted practices. However, the authors, editors, and publisher are not responsible for errors or omissions or for any consequences from application of the information in this book and make no warranty, express or implied, with respect to the contents of the publication.

The authors, editors, and publisher have exerted every effort to ensure that drug selection and dosage set forth in this text are in accordance with current recommendations and practice at the time of publication. However, in view of ongoing research, changes in government regulations, and the constant flow of information relating to drug therapy and drug reactions, the reader is urged to check the package insert for each drug for any change in indications and dosage and for added warnings and precautions. This is particularly important when the recommended agent is a new or infrequently employed drug.

Some drugs and medical devices presented in this publication have Food and Drug Administration (FDA) clearance for limited use in restricted research settings. It is the responsibility of the health care provider to ascertain the FDA status of each drug or device planned for use in their clinical practice.

Who Was "Rypins"?

D r. Harold Rypins (1892–1939) was the founding editor of what is now known as the RYPINS' series of review books. Originally published under the title *Medical State Board Examinations,* the first edition was published by J. B. Lippincott Company in 1933. Dr. Rypins edited subsequent editions of the book in 1935, 1937, and 1939 before his death that year. The series that he began has since become the longest-running and most successful publication of its kind, having served as an invaluable tool in the training of generations of medical students. Dr. Rypins was a member of the faculty of Albany Medical College in Albany, New York, and also served as Secretary of the New York State Board of Medical Examiners. His legacy to medical education flourishes today in the highly successful *Rypins' Basic Sciences Review* and *Rypins' Clinical Sciences Review,* now in the 17th editions, and in the *Rypins' Intensive Reviews* series of subject review volumes. We at Lippincott Williams & Wilkins Publishers take pride in this continuing success.

—*The Publisher*

▼ Series Preface

These are indeed very exciting times in medicine. Having made this statement, one's thoughts immediately reflect about the major changes that are occurring in our overall healthcare delivery system, utilization-review and shortened hospitalizations, issues concerning quality assurance, ambulatory surgical procedures and medical clearances, and the impact of managed care on the practice of internal medicine and primary care. Each of these issues has had a considerable impact on the approach to the patient and on the practice of medicine.

But even more mind-boggling than the foregoing changes are the dramatic changes imposed on the practice of medicine by fundamental conceptual scientific innovations engendered by advances in basic science that no doubt will affect medical practice of the immediate future. Indeed, much of what we thought of as having a potential impact on the practice of medicine of the future has already been perceived. One need only take a cursory look at our weekly medical journals to realize that we are practicing "tomorrow's medicine today." And consider that the goal a few years ago of actually describing the human genome is now near reality.

Reflect, then, for a moment on our current thinking about genetics, molecular biology, cellular immunology, and other areas that have impacted upon our current understanding of the underlying mechanisms of the pathophysiological concepts of disease. Moreover, paralleling these innovations have been remarkable advances in the so-called "high tech" and "gee-whiz" aspects of how we diagnose disease and treat patients. We can now think with much greater perspective about the dimensions of more specific biologic diagnoses concerned with molecular perturbations; gene therapy not only affecting genetic but oncological disease; more specific pharmacotherapy involving highly specific receptor inhibition, alterations of intracellular signal transduction, manipulations of cellular protein synthesis; immunosuppresive therapy not only with respect to organ transplantations but also of autoimmune and other immune-related disease; and therapeutic means for manipulating organ remodeling or the intravascular placement of stents. Each of these concepts has become inculcated into our everyday medical practice within the past decade. The reason why these changes have so rapidly promoted an upheaval in medical practice is continuing medical education, a constant awareness of the current medical literature, and a thirst for new knowledge.

To assist the student and practitioner in the review process, the publisher and I have initiated a new approach in the publication of *Rypins' Basic Sciences Review* and *Rypins' Clinical Sciences Review*. Thus, when I assumed responsibility to edit this long-standing board review series with the 13th edition of the textbook (first published in 1931), it was with a feeling of great excitement. I perceived that great changes would be coming to medicine, and I believed that this would be one ideal means of not only facing these changes head on but also for me personally to cope and keep up with these changes. Over the subsequent editions, this confidence was reassured and rewarded. The presentation for the updating of medical information was tremendously enhanced by the substitution of new authors, as the former authority "standbys" stepped down or retired from our faculty. Each of the authors who continue to be selected for maintaining the character of our textbook is an authority in his or her respective area and has had considerable pedagogic and formal examination experience. One dramatic recent example of the changes in author replacement just came about with the 17th edition. When I invited Dr. Peter Goldblatt to participate in the authorship of the pathology chapter of the textbook, his answer was "what goes around, comes around." You see, Dr. Goldblatt's father, Dr. Harry Goldblatt, a major contributor to the history of hypertensive disease, was the first author of the pathology chapter in 1931. What a satisfying experience for me personally. Other less human changes in our format came with the establishment of two soft cover volumes, the current basic and clinical sciences review volumes, replacing the single volume text of earlier years. Soon, a third supplementary volume concerned with questions and answers for the basic science volume appeared. Accompanying these more obvious changes was the constant updating of the knowledge base of each of the chapters, and this continues on into the present 17th edition.

And now we have introduced another major innovation in our presentation of the basic and clinical sciences reviews. This change is evidenced by the introduction of the *Rypins' Intensive Reviews* series, along with the 17th edition of *Rypins' Basic Sciences Review, Rypins' Clinical Sciences Review,* and the *Questions and Answers* third volume. These volumes are written to be used separately from the parent textbook. Each not only contains the material published in the respective chapters of the textbook, but is considerably "fleshed out" in the discussion, tables, figures, and questions and answers. Thus, the *Rypins' Intensive Reviews* series serves as an important supplement to the overall review process and also provides a study guide for those already in practice in preparing for specific specialty board certification and recertification examinations.

Therefore, with continued confidence and excitement, I am pleased to present these innovations in review experience for your consideration. As in the past, I look forward to learning of your comments and suggestions. In doing so, we continue to look forward to our continued growth and acceptance of the *Rypins'* review experience.

Edward D. Frohlich, MD, MACP, FACC

▼
Preface

Over the past 20 years, medicine has seen the field of community health and clinical epidemiology progress from esoteric subjects to mainstream concerns. The phenomena of Health Maintenance Organizations (HMOs) and other forms of managed care have focused even more the attention of health administrators, physicians, and patients on "population medicine." The areas of epidemiology and biostatistics have become the "basic sciences" of community medicine. All newly trained physicians, regardless of discipline, will need to be familiar with these areas to practice population medicine and to be able to interpret the medical literature where, increasingly, clinical trials are the primary methodology. This book is designed for medical students as an introduction to the most important basic concepts of community medicine. This is not a comprehensive textbook, but rather an overall review of the main topics in public health and community medicine. The questions at the end of the book are written in the United States Medical Licensing Examination (USMLE) format. Answering the questions and reading the answers and discussions will provide additional understanding of the field.

▼

Introduction

Preparing for USMLE

THE NATIONAL BOARD OF MEDICAL EXAMINERS

For years the National Board examinations have served as an index of the medical education of the period and have strongly influenced higher educational standards in each of the medical sciences. The Diploma of the National Board is accepted by 47 state licensing authorities, the District of Columbia, and the Commonwealth of Puerto Rico in lieu of the examination usually required for licensure and is recognized in the American Medical Directory by the letters DNB following the name of the physician holding National Board certification.

The National Board of Medical Examiners (NBME) has been a leader in developing new and more reliable techniques of testing, not only for knowledge in all medical fields but also for clinical competence and fitness to practice. In recent years, too, a number of medical schools, several specialty certifying boards, professional medical societies organized to encourage their members to keep abreast of progress in medicine, and other professional qualifying agencies have called upon the National Board's professional staff for advice or for the actual preparation of tests to be employed in evaluating medical knowledge, effectiveness of teaching and professional competence in certain medical fields. In all cases, advantage has been taken of the validity and effectiveness of the objective, multiple-choice type of examination, a technique the National Board has played an important role in bringing to its present state of perfection and discriminatory effectiveness.

The National Board of Medical Examiners examination is now much like that for the United States Medical Licensing Examination (USMLE). The examinations of the National Board has become recognized as the most comprehensive test of knowledge of the medical sciences and their clinical application produced in this country. Like the USMLE, the National Board has contracted with the Sylvan Learning Centers to provide individual examinations for the candidate on an individual basis and the questions follow the same concept of random allocation of questions in groups of 50. The candidate is given the opportunity to skip over questions in that group of 50 and the provision to return to any of the skipped questions before proceeding on to the next group of 50. The advantages of these questions are the same as those for the USMLE and the students have reported that, under this format, they are less "stressed out" and better able to cope with the examination.

As outlined in the 1999 USMLE Bulletin of Information on Computer-based Testing (CBT), all medical students or graduates of a United States or Canadian medical school accredited by the Liaison Committee on Medical Education (or by the American Osteopathic Association) should contact the NBME for application materials to sit for the National Board examinations. For graduates of both U.S. and foreign medical schools, those individuals interested in obtaining the up-to-the-minute information should contact the National Board of Medical Examiners at 3750 Market Street, Philadelphia, PA 19104. The telephone number of the NBME is (215)590-9500.

UNITED STATES MEDICAL LICENSING EXAMINATION (USMLE)

In August 1991 the Federation of State Medical Boards (FSMB) and the NBME agreed to replace their respective examinations, the FLEX and NBME, with a new examination, the United States Medical Licensing Examination (USMLE). This examination will provide a common means for evaluating all applicants for medical licensure. It appears that this development in medical licensure will at last satisfy the needs for state medical boards licensure, the national medical board licensure, and licensure examinations for foreign medical graduates. This is because the 1991 agreement provides for a composite committee that equally represents both organizations (the FSMB and NBME) as well as a jointly appointed public member and a representative of the Educational Council for Foreign Medical Graduates (ECFMG).

As indicated in the USMLE announcement, "It is expected that students who enrolled in U.S. medical schools in the fall of 1990 or later and foreign medical graduates applying for ECFMG examinations beginning in 1993 will have access only to USMLE for purposes of licensure." The phaseout of the last regular examinations for licensure was completed in December 1994.

The new USMLE is administered in three steps. Step 1 focuses on fundamental basic biomedical science concepts, with particular emphasis on "principles and mechanisms underlying disease and modes of therapy." Step 2 is related to the clinical sciences, with examination on material necessary to practice medicine in a supervised setting. Step 3 is designed to focus on "aspects of biomedical and clinical science essential for the unsupervised practice of medicine."

Today Step 1 and Step 2 examinations are set up and scored as total comprehensive objective tests in the basic sciences and clinical sciences, respectively. The format of each part is no longer subject-oriented, that is, separated into sections specifically labeled Anatomy, Pathology, Medicine, Surgery, and so forth. Subject labels are therefore missing, and in each part questions from the different fields are intermixed or integrated so that the subject origin of any individual question is not immediately apparent, although it is known by the National Board office. Therefore, if necessary, individual subject grades can be extracted.

Very recently, the National Board of Medical Examiners contracted with Sylvan Prometric, a division of Sylvan Learning Systems, to provide scheduling and test centers for the USMLE for all applicants who have registered with the Educational Commission for Foreign Medical Graduates (ECFMG) and who are familiar with the 1999 ECFMG Information Booklet for Computer-based Testing (CBT). These examinations are given at the Sylvan technology centers around the United States and elsewhere around the world. The applicant can arrange to take his/her one-day examination at a mutually convenient time under the direct supervision of that Sylvan center. The student sits at his/her own assigned computer at the Center to proceed with the randomly assigned questions. The questions given to each student are similar among students, but each test is unique.

As in the past, the Step 1 test includes questions in anatomy, biochemistry, microbiology, pathology, pharmacology, physiology, and the behavioral sciences. Questions in such areas as molecular biology, cell biology, and genetics are included, as well as questions which are designed to test the "candidates recognition of the similarity or dissimilarity of disease, drugs, and physiologic, behavioral, or pathologic processes." Problems are presented in narrative, tabular, or graphic format, followed by questions designed to assess the candidate's knowledge and comprehension of the situation that is described.

Step 2 includes questions in internal medicine, obstetrics and gynecology, pediatrics, preventive medicine and public health, psychiatry, and surgery. The style of the questions is similar to Step 1. A broad spectrum of knowledge is covered in each of the clinical fields. In addition to individual questions, specific clinical problems are presented in the form of patient histories, physical examinations, charts, roentgenograms, electrocardiograms, photographs of gross and microscopic pathologic specimens, laboratory data, and the like. The candidate must answer questions relating to the interpretation of the data presented and their relationship to the clinical problems. The questions are "designed to explore the extent of the candidate's knowledge of clinical situations, and to test his/her ability to bring information from many different clinical and basic science areas to bear upon these situations."

In both the Step 1 and 2 examinations, the student selects questions in groups of 50. The format permits the student to proceed to the next question (or return to unanswered questions) within that group of those 50 questions under consideration. Then, after completing one group of 50 questions, the student then proceeds to another 50 questions (and so on) until the examination is completed. After each group of 50 questions is completed, however, the student cannot return to a previous grouping. All questions in both Step 1 and Step 2 are clinically oriented and require one best answer.

The style and format of this examination is designed to prevent any breach of confidentiality of the examination, and the overall procedure is exceedingly well-controlled in a highly disciplined environment.

This type of interdisciplinary examination and the method of scoring the entire test as a unit have definite advantages, especially in view of the changing curricula in medical schools. The former type of rigid, almost standardized, curriculum, with its emphasis on specific subjects and a specified number of hours in each, has been replaced by a more liberal, open-ended curriculum, permitting emphasis in one or more fields and corresponding deemphasis in others. The result has been rather wide variations in the totality of education in different medical schools. Thus, the scoring of these tests as a whole permits accommodation to this variability in the curricula of different schools. Within the total score, weakness in one subject that has received relatively little emphasis in a given school may be balanced by strength in other subjects.

The rationale for this type of comprehensive examination as replacement for the traditional department-oriented examination in the basic sciences and the clinical sciences is given in the National Board Examiner:

The student, as he [or she] confronts these examinations, must abandon the idea of "thinking like a physiologist" in answering a question labeled "physiology" or "thinking like a surgeon" in answering a question labeled "surgery." The one question may have been written by a biochemist or a pharmacologist; the other question may have been written by an internist or a pediatrician. The pattern of these examinations will direct the student to thinking more broadly of the basic sciences in Step 1 and to thinking of patients and their problems in Step 2.

Until a few years ago, the Part I examination could not be taken until the work of the second year in medical school had been completed, and the Part II test was given only to students who had completed the major part of the fourth year. Now students, if they feel they are ready, may be admitted to any regularly scheduled Step 1 or Step 2 examination during any year of their medical course without prerequisite completion of specified courses or chronologic periods of study. Thus, emphasis is placed on the acquisition of knowledge and competence rather than the completion of predetermined periods.

Candidates are eligible for Step 3 after they have passed Steps 1 and 2, have received the M.D. degree from an approved medical school in the United States or Canada, and subsequent to the receipt of the M.D. degree, have served at least six months in an approved hospital internship or residency. Under certain circumstances, consideration may be given to other types of graduate training provided they meet with the approval of the National Board. After passing the Step 3 examination, candidates will receive their Diplomas as of the date of the satisfactory completion of an internship or residency program. If candidates have completed the approved hospital training prior to completion of Step 3, they will receive certification as of the date of the successful completion of Step 3.

At the time of this publication, the details for the Step 3 part of the USMLE are not certain. The applicant for this part of the examination is recommended to communicate directly with ECFMG for these details.

QUESTIONS

Over the years, many different forms of objective questions have been devised to test not only medical knowledge but also those subtler qualities of discrimination, judgment, and reasoning. Certain types of questions may test an individual's recognition of the similarity or dissimilarity of diseases, drugs, and physiologic or pathologic processes. Other questions test judgment as to cause and effect or the lack of causal relationships. Case histories or patient problems are used to simulate the experience of a physician confronted with a diagnostic problem; a series of questions then tests the individual's understanding of related aspects of the case, such as signs and symptoms, associated laboratory findings, treatment, complications, and prognosis. Case-history questions are set up purposely to place emphasis on correct diagnosis within a context comparable with the experience of actual practice.

It is apparent from recent certification and board examinations that the examiners are devoting more attention in their construction of questions to more practical means of testing basic and clinical knowledge. This greater realism in testing relates to an increasingly interdisciplinary approach toward fundamental material and to the direct relevance accorded practical clinical problems. These more recent approaches to questions have been incorporated into this review series.

Of course, the new approaches to testing add to the difficulty experienced by the student or physician preparing for board or certification examinations. With this in mind, the author of this review is acutely aware not only of the interrelationships of fundamental information within the basic science disciplines and their clinical implications but also of the necessity to present this material clearly and concisely despite its complexity. For this reason, the questions are devised to test knowledge of specific material within the text and identify areas for more intensive study, if necessary. Also, those preparing for examinations must be aware of the interdisciplinary nature of fundamental clinical material, the common multifactorial characteristics of disease mechanisms, and the necessity to shift back and forth from one discipline to another in order to appreciate the less than clear-cut nature separating the pedagogic disciplines.

The different types of questions that may be used on examinations include the completion-type question, where the individual must select one best answer among a number of possible choices, most often five, although there may be three or four; the completion-type question in the negative form, where all but one of the choices is correct and words such as *except* or *least* appear in the question; the true-false type of question, which tests an understanding of cause and effect in relationship to medicine; the multiple true-false type, in which the question may have one, several, or all correct choices; one matching-type question, which tests association and relatedness and uses four choices, two of which use the word, *both* or *neither;* another matching-type question that uses anywhere from three to twenty-six choices and may have more than one correct answer; and, as noted above, the patient-oriented question, which is written around a case and may have several questions included as a group or set.

For further detailed information concerning developments in the evolution of the examination process for medical licensure (for graduates of both U.S. and foreign medical schools), those interested should contact the National Board of Medical Examiners at 3750 Market Street, Philadelphia, PA 19104, USA; telephone number (215)590–9500.

FIVE POINTS TO REMEMBER

In order for the candidate to maximize chances for passing these examinations, a few common sense strategies or guidelines should be kept in mind.

First, it is imperative to prepare thoroughly for the examination. Know well the types of questions to be presented and the pedagogic areas of particular weakness, and devote more preparatory study time to these areas of weakness. Do not use too much time restudying areas in which there is a feeling of great confidence and do not leave unexplored those areas in which there is less confidence. Finally, be well rested before the test and, if possible, avoid traveling to the city of testing that morning or late the evening before.

Second, know well the format of the examination and the instructions before becoming immersed in the challenge at hand. This information can be obtained from many published texts and brochures or directly from the testing service (National Board of Medical Examiners, 3750 Market Street, Philadelphia, PA 19104;

telephone (215) 590–9500). In addition, many available texts and self-assessment types of examination are valuable for practice.

Third, know well the overall time allotted for the examination and its components and the scope of the test to be faced. These may be learned by a rapid review of the examination itself. Then, proceed with the test at a careful, deliberate, and steady pace without spending an inordinate amount of time on any single question.

Fourth, if a question is particularly disturbing, note appropriately the question and return to this point later. Don't compromise yourself by so concentrating on a likely "loser" that several "winners" are eliminated because of inadequate time. One way to save this time on a particular "stickler" is to play your initial choice; your chances of a correct answer are always best with your first impression. If there is no initial choice, reread the question.

Fifth, allow adequate time to review answers, to return to the questions that were unanswered for later attention.

There is nothing magical about these five points. They are simple and just make common sense. If you have prepared well, have gotten a good night's sleep, have eaten a good breakfast, and follow the preceding five points, the chances are that you will not have to return for a second go-around.

Edward D. Frohlich, MD, MACP, FACC

Series Acknowledgments

In no other writing experience is one more dependent on others than in a textbook, especially a textbook that provides a broad review for the student and fellow practitioner. In this spirit, I am truly indebted to all who have contributed to our past and current understanding of the fundamental and clinical aspects related to the practice of medicine. No one individual ever provides the singular "breakthrough" so frequently attributed as such by the news media. Knowledge develops and grows as a result of continuing and exciting contributions of research from all disciplines, academic institutions, and nations. Clearly, outstanding investigators have been credited for major contributions, but those with true and understanding humility are quick to attribute the preceding input of knowledge by others to the growing body of knowledge. In this spirit, we acknowledge the long list of contributors to medicine over the generations. We also acknowledge that in no century has man so exceeded the sheer volume of these advances than in the twentieth century. Indeed, it has been said by many that the sum of new knowledge over the past 50 years has most likely exceeded all that had been contributed in the prior years.

With this spirit of more universal acknowledgment, I wish to recognize personally the interest, support, and suggestions made by my colleagues in my institution and elsewhere. I specifically refer to those people from my institution who were of particular help and are listed at the outset of the internal medicine volume. But, in addition to these colleagues, I want to express my deep appreciation to my institution and clinic for providing the opportunity and ambience to maintain and continue these academic pursuits. As I have often said, the primary mission of a school of medicine is that of education and research; the care of patients, a long secondary mission to ensure the conduct of the primary goal, has now also become a primary commitment in these more pragmatic times. In contrast, the primary mission of the major multidisciplinary clinics has been the care of patients, with education and research assuming secondary roles as these commitments become affordable. It is this distinction that sets the multispecialty clinic apart from other modes of medical practice.

Over and above a personal commitment and drive to assure publication of a textbook such as this is the tremendous support and loyalty of a hard-working and dedicated office staff. To this end, I am tremendously grateful and indebted to Mrs. Lillian Buffa and Mrs. Caramia Fairchild. Their long hours of unselfish work on my behalf and to satisfy their own interest in participating in this major educational effort is appreciated to no end. I am personally deeply honored and thankful for their important roles in the publication of the Rypins' series.

Words of appreciation must be extended to the staff of the Lippincott–Raven, now Lippincott Williams & Wilkins, Publishers. It is more than 25 years since I have become associated with this publishing house, one of the first to be established in our nation. Over these years, I have worked closely with Mr. Richard Winters, not only with the Rypins' editions but also with other textbooks. His has been a labor of commitment, interest, and full support—not only because of his responsibility to his institution, but also because of the excitement of the publishing of new knowledge. In recent years, we discussed at length the merits of adding the intensive review supplements to the parent textbook and together we worked out the details that have become the substance of our present "joint venture." Moreover, together we are willing to make the necessary changes to assure the intellectual success of this series. To this end, we are delighted to include a new member of our team effort, Ms. Susan Kelly. She joined our cause to ensure that the format of questions, the reference process of answers to those questions within the text itself, and the editorial process involved be natural and clear to our readers. I am grateful for each of these facets of the overall publication process.

Not the least is my everlasting love and appreciation to my family. I am particularly indebted to my parents who inculcated in me at a very early age the love of education, the respect for study and hard work, and the honor for those who share these values. In this regard, it would have been impossible for me to accomplish any of my academic pursuits without the love, inspiration, and continued support of my wife, Sherry. Not only has she maintained the personal encouragement to initiate and continue with these labors of love, but she has sustained and supported our family and home life so that these activities could be encouraged. Hopefully, these pursuits have not detracted from the development and love of our children, Margie, Bruce, and Lara. I assume that this has not occurred; we are so very proud that each is personally committed to education and research. How satisfying it is to realize that these ideals remain a familial characteristic.

Edward D. Frohlich, MD, MACP, FACC
New Orleans, Louisiana

Acknowledgments

This book was made possible with the technical assistance of Tom Lawrence. I would also like to thank Karen Margolis, M.D., M.P.H, John Flack, M.D., M.P.H, and Nancy J. Mendelsohn, M.D., for assistance in writing this book.

Contents

CONTENTS

Chapter 5

Evidence-Based Medicine   53

Chapter 6

Managed Care   55

Chapter 7

Health Services Research   59

Chapter 8

Ethnicity   63

Chapter 9

High Priority Areas for Community Medicine   67

Community Health Questions   91

Community Health Answers and Discussion   131

Community Health Must-Know Topics   143

Index   145

Chapter 1

Introduction to Public Health and Community Medicine

To the medical student just finishing 4 years of school and eager to start a residency working with "real patients," the arena of public health usually holds little charm. To these students (and most practicing physicians), the primary focus is *individual patient care;* after all, isn't that what the 4 years of didactic and clinical apprenticeship in medical school pointed toward? During the years of clinical education, mentors emphasize establishing a differential diagnosis and, by exclusion and deductive reasoning, arriving at the diagnosis. Less attention is given to selecting the appropriate treatments and ensuring adherence to those treatments; even less is given to achieving adequate follow-up and continuity of care.

Practicing physicians rightfully focus on diagnosis and individual patient care as their main concern; however, much is lost by not including the public health and community medicine perspective as well. When a physician diagnoses a condition, it has usually been preceded by years or even decades of exposures that caused the disease; the condition may have existed for many additional years in the subacute asymptomatic state. Although it is gratifying to make the correct diagnosis at the end stage of a disease, treatment at that point in the natural history of the disease is often, at best, palliative and, at worst, harmful. Including a public health perspective in medical teaching encourages physicians to get more involved in much earlier stages of the disease and to help prevent disease from developing. Because the early stage of disease begins in the community, the community is the appropriate focus of this involvement.

In addition to diagnosis, contemporary physicians must also be able to evaluate and select appropriate treatments. Modern medical treatments, although impressive, may have significant potential for harm; therefore, careful evaluation of new therapies is needed. A primary tool for evaluating new therapies is the **randomized clinical trial**. To properly evaluate results of such a trial, physicians need to understand the design, method, and analysis of the trial.

Community medicine bridges the gap between clinical medicine and public health, dealing with people and patients within the community. This text covers basic concepts of public health and community medicine, giving a vital perspective not only to those who expect to devote themselves to research in prevention and treatment of disease in large populations but also to those whose focus will be the practice of individual patient care.

For most physicians who see only individual patients, it is difficult to appreciate the potential for prevention in community-based interventions. Physicians may assume that, to prevent disease in a patient, major changes in lifestyle (e.g., smoking cessation and weight loss) are necessary for the patient to benefit. They may become skeptical that these changes are possible after seeing the difficulties that many patients and families undergo in trying to make major lifestyle changes. They may doubt that moderate changes in behavior will lower risk significantly and justify the disruptions and considerable effort made by the patient to make the changes. They may be aware, for example, that the difficult task of cutting sodium intake by 50 mEq, or about one third, might result in a 2- to 3-mmHg reduction in diastolic pressure, an improvement that seems small when compared to a 10-mmHg reduction achieved more easily with drugs. Most physicians are not enthusiastic about prevention when observations of the individual provide their sole basis for judgment.

A different view of prevention arises, however, when another paradigm is considered—the **population perspective,** which looks at trends within the community as a whole. Even though high-risk patients in the population (e.g., persons with severe hypertension or hypercholesteremia, or heavy cigarette smokers) have the greatest *absolute risk* for contracting disease, most of the *actual cases* of disease (e.g., deaths, heart attacks, and strokes) are found in persons whose health is considered average or above-average but not necessarily "abnormal" by conventional medical standards. Thus, if this very large, lower risk population can change its distribution of risk factor only slightly, then the amount of disease that could be prevented in the community is substantial. Figure 1-1 uses serum cholesterol levels as

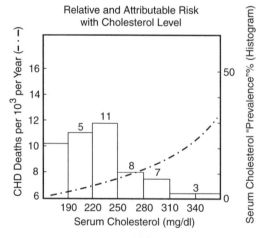

Figure 1-1.
Serum cholesterol. (Blackburn H. Coronary Risk Factors—How to Evaluate Them. *Eur J Cardiol* 1975;2:252.)

an example to illustrate this phenomenon. Furthermore, if only a small change in average blood pressure (approximately 2 mmHg systolic) could be achieved through the efforts of physicians, schools, media, and volunteer organizations working in conjunction to lower sodium and weight in the community as a whole, then a substantial percentage of cases of stroke and heart attack could be prevented. If physicians take into account both the individual patient and the population perspective, they can expect to improve greatly their ability to prevent disease and to provide treatment within their communities.

Chapter 2

Health Statistics

Health has been defined in many ways. Many people think of health as the absence of disease; however, it is less than precise to define something by what it is not. The World Health Organization (WHO) defined health in 1948 as "a state of complete physical, mental, and social well-being, and not merely the absence of disease or infirmity."

Clear definition is the first step in measurement, setting limits that tell whether subjects fall within or outside of the delimiters. Measurement then goes further to indicate more precisely where a subject falls along a scale. Most devices used to measure public health have evolved from the fields of health statistics, biometry, and epidemiology.

Because the population is the base for most health statistics, complete enumeration of the population is important. In the first year of each decade, the US Census Bureau conducts a national census to provide this information. The estimates made for intermediate years are sufficiently reliable for the purposes of most research, but historically they have missed many minority and low socioeconomic patients. Consideration is being given to using a complete count of random subgroups for the year 2000 census. This approach is less likely to miss important subgroups.

Population trends in the United States differ from those in developing countries where controlling population growth is difficult. Family planning activities are adopted more slowly, but lifesaving techniques that took more advanced countries decades to develop take only a few years to adopt. In most developing countries, then, birth rates are out of proportion to the more rapid decrease in death rates.

No form of life can continue to multiply without eventually coming to terms with its environment. Thus, the rate of human population growth must inevitably slow down and level off. The major questions are when, at what levels, and at what cost to the public health will this occur? Predictions regarded as reasonable in the mid-1980s suggest that the world population will continue to expand through the first half of the 21st century (Figure 2-1).

In contrast to population figures, which form the denominators of most health statistics, vital facts concerning birth rates, morbidity, and numbers of deaths form the numerators. Registration of births and deaths by the departments of health of the various states is required throughout the United States. Attending physicians are re-

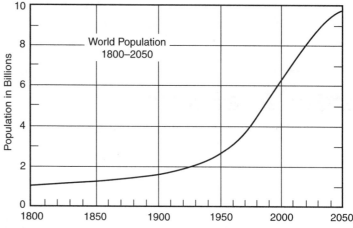

Figure 2-1.
Estimates of the world population in billions, 1800 to 2050.

sponsible for filing birth certificates with local registrars, and funeral directors are responsible for filing death and stillbirth certificates.

In the internationally agreed-upon form of the death certificate, Part I emphasizes the underlying cause of death as determined by the certifying physician. Because many older patients who die have multiple diseases, the way in which physicians select the underlying cause of death may have an important effect on reported time trends in death rates. There is good evidence that certain swings in death rates in recent decades relate more to changes in diagnostic trends among physicians than to true changes in incidence of diseases. To compensate for such variations, the United States is beginning to attempt to record and analyze all causes on the death certificate rather than only the underlying cause.

DEATH CERTIFICATION/DEATH RATES

For more than 50 years, the United States has had mandatory standardized certification of all deaths. It is the physician's duty to fill out death certificates and ascribe an immediate cause of death as a consequence of a specific disease. Death certificates are collected locally and forwarded to state health departments, where records are kept and summary data are developed. Death certificates are coded for specific diseases by nosologists using a standard International Classification of Diseases System (ICDS). Data tapes from state health departments are sent to the National Center for Health Statistics (NCHS), where national summary data are compiled and periodically published. Current death certification is virtually 100% complete in the United States, Canada, and Europe; however, most developing countries do not have adequate systems for certifying deaths, and data from such countries are far from accurate.

The primary causes of death in the United States have changed dramatically since 1900 when infectious diseases were by far the most common cause of death (Table 2-1). Because of improved hygiene and medical care, infectious diseases currently account for a relatively small percentage of total deaths, although several emerging infectious outbreaks are being reported. This is thought to be related to the widespread overprescription of antibiotics. In 1998, chronic diseases such as heart disease and stroke as well as cancer together are responsible for about one half of all deaths.

Although death certification is useful and allows the tracking of disease incidence and prevalence over time, there are problems with validity. Studies comparing autopsy death ascertainment with death certifications show that less than 10% of deaths are autopsied. There is some discrepancy between death certification and autopsy; for example, cardiovascular diseases tend to be somewhat overestimated by death certification compared to autopsy, whereas cancer deaths are more accurately reflected. Nevertheless, the system works well to reflect change of disease incidence over time and to serve as an early warning system for new disease developments such as outbreaks of influenza or acquired immunodeficiency syndrome (AIDS).

Two indices are often used to describe the frequency of a disease in the population:

1. **Incidence rate**—the number of new cases of the disease occurring over an interval of time in the population. Incidence rate is often adjusted for age, race, and gender distribution of the specified population so that figures from relatively young and relatively old groups can be compared.
2. **Prevalence rate**—the number of cases of the disease in the population present at one point or cross section in time.

TABLE 2-1.

Primary Causes of Death

1900	1994
Pneumonia, 11.7%	Heart diseases, 32.1%
Tuberculosis, 11.3%	Cancer, 23.5%
Diarrhea and enteritis, 8.3%	Stroke, 6.8%
Heart diseases, 8.0%	Bronchitis and emphysema, 4.5%
Stroke, 6.2%	Injuries, 3.9%
Liver disease, 5.1%	Pneumonia and influenza, 3.6%
Injuries, 4.2%	Diabetes, 2.4%
Cancer, 3.7%	HIV Infection, 1.8%
Senility, 2.9%	Suicide, 1.4%
Diphtheria, 2.3%	Chronic liver disease, 1.1%

Percentage of all deaths.

Sources: Centers for Disease Control and Prevention, National Center for Health Statistics.

Both incidence and prevalence rates are usually expressed as cases per 100,000 population. These figures are often made specific for age, gender, and race. The longer the duration of illness, the greater the number of cases in the population at any point in time. Thus, a high prevalence rate may reflect a high incidence rate, a long duration of illness, or both. Prevalence reflects a community photograph of disease at one moment in time. When illness is rare, the larger prevalence ratio is more easily understood and studied than is the smaller incidence rate.

Generally, cause of death should be reported in accordance with the disease classification developed by the International Statistical Classification of Diseases, Injuries, and Causes of Death, which is distributed by the WHO. The ninth revision of this WHO publication, first used in the United States for 1979 death statistics, produced some artificial changes in death rates between 1978 and 1979. Such changes in classification of causes of death must be taken into account when interpreting the significance of death rates. In addition to providing important data on health problems, the death certificate is used for legal purposes such as the settlement of estates and insurance claims.

The mortality statistics compiled from the death registrations are usually expressed as rates, including

- crude death rates
- specific death rates
- infant mortality rates
- maternal mortality rates

Crude Death Rate

The **crude death rate** is formed by the number of deaths in a calendar year per 1,000 population at the middle of that year. After having decreased rapidly between 1930 and 1950, the crude death rate for the United States changed little in the 1950s and 1960s and then decreased again in the 1970s. In the United States, in 1987, the rate was 8.7/1,000 (Figure 2-2). Crude death rates in the United States reflect the pattern of deaths primarily in the older population, and in each year they also show a seasonal pattern, with winter highs and summer lows (Figure 2-3). Crude death rates decrease more swiftly in developing countries, however, wherein older age groups form a smaller proportion of the total population. In the United States, death rates also decline more steeply when adjusted for the increasing age of the total population (see Figure 2-2).

Specific Death Rate

Specific death rates are calculated for certain groups because the crude death rate is much affected by age, gender, ethnic group, and marital and socioeconomic differences in the population being studied. One example is the **age-specific death rate,** which is formed by

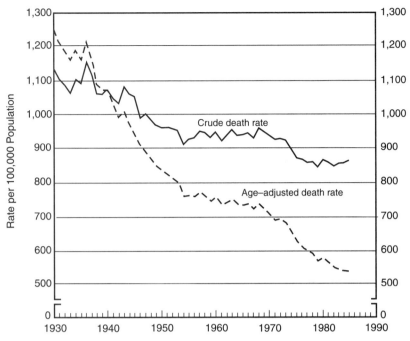

Figure 2-2.
Crude and age-adjusted death rates per 100,000 US population, 1930 to 1985. The crude rate hides part of the decline in deaths because it does not adjust for the expanding elderly population.

the number of deaths in a specific age group in a given year per 1,000 population at that specified age. In any given year, however, age-specific rates are low until age 30 years, after which they increase markedly into older ages. A population with a high proportion of elderly persons has a high crude death rate. To compare mortality rates in the same country in different years, standardized procedures are used to correct for changing age distributions. These calculations produce an **age-adjusted death rate,** which declines more steeply for the United States than the crude death rate does (see Figure 2-2). At every age, the adjusted rates have decreased since 1900.

In the United States, at almost every age, mortality rate in women is lower than in men; this is not the case in most developing countries where complications of childbirth occurring under adverse conditions increase the mortality rates of women of reproductive age.

Death rates in the United States are higher in men than in women for coronary heart disease, chronic obstructive lung disease, lung cancer, and accidents. One cause of death for which **death rates have become similar in men and women is diabetes mellitus;** previously, the death rate was higher in women. Age-specific death rates have decreased more for women than for men in the United States and more for whites than for African Americans. Socioeconomic factors and perhaps inferior health care among African Americans are believed to be partly responsible for this latter difference.

Specific death rates are also developed for gender, race, marital status, and other factors. At each age, for example, death rates among the married population are lower than among the unmarried

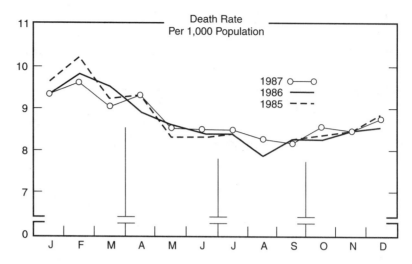

Figure 2-3.
Seasonal change in crude death rates per 1000 US population, by month of calendar years 1985, 1986, and 1987.

population; this finding is partly explained by the likelihood that persons who marry are already more healthy than those who do not, but other factors may also play a role.

Disease-specific death rates are widely used in most developed countries. Each rate is the number of deaths from a given disease during the year per 100,000 population. Until the 1980s, the rates were based on the diagnosis that the attending physician stated to be the underlying cause of death. The death rate for a particular disease was assumed to reflect the size of the threat to public health from that condition.

Infant Mortality Rate

The **infant mortality rate** is the number of deaths among children younger than 1 year of age in a given year per 1,000 live births in the same year. Rates for African Americans are consistently higher than rates for whites. The infant mortality rate was formerly regarded as a good (perhaps the best) measure of the effectiveness of public health programs, wherein a good public health program correlated to a decrease in infant mortality rate and with the infant mortality rate being sensitive to changes in society, including improvements in health care. However, it seems likely that reductions in infant mortality rates exaggerate the effectiveness of environmental health, communicable disease, and maternal and child health programs in former years. They do not reflect well on current efforts to treat chronic disease, mental illness, and other problems of the older population. Infant mortality rates are lower in many other developed countries than they are in the United States. It seems clear that certain differences are real and not caused artificially by data manipulation. Nevertheless, it is difficult to separate the effect of improved medical care from that of socioeconomic improvements and nutritional advances. The neonatal death rate, part of the infant mortality rate based on deaths occurring in the first 4 weeks of life, has come to be viewed by some as the better measure of health care effects. Thus, the debate over the value of infant mortality rates in assessing the health of populations has been vigorous in the United States.

Maternal Mortality Rate

The **maternal mortality rate** is determined by the number of deaths attributed to puerperal causes in a given year per 1,000 live births in the same year. Like the infant mortality rate in the United States, this rate is decreasing more slowly and is considerably higher for non-whites than for whites. **Hypertensive disease of pregnancy is the largest single cause of maternal death.**

Leading Causes of Death

The leading causes of death have changed radically since 1900. At the beginning of the 20th century, infections such as tuberculosis, influenza, and pneumonia were the dominant causes of death. Currently, noninfectious chronic diseases are dominant, with cardiovascular disease and cancer being the major causes of death, making up approximately 50% and 22% of all causes of death, respectively. Those who set priorities for disease control programs for society, however, must also consider the average age of death and the likelihood of success in disease prevention when setting policies for public health.

Another commonly used measure of health is **life expectancy.** Although the average expectation of life is sometimes advocated as a "positive" measure of health—the higher the figure, the better the public health—life expectancy is basically determined by the death rates of the population involved. The lower the subsequent death rates, the higher is the expectation of life. It is hard to argue convincingly that the expectation of life measures something different from the force of mortality. Figure 2-4 shows that life expectancy at birth has slowly increased in recent decades. It is consistently higher for women than for men.

Professionals interested in disease prevention and health promotion have been concerned that disease and death have been overemphasized as measures of public health. For this and other reasons, age-specific death rates are used to calculate the likelihood of surviving and the average years of life remaining at any given age. The results of these life table calculations are illustrated in Table 2-2, based on the death rates occurring in the United States in 1980. More detailed life tables form the statistical basis for the work of life insurance companies. The same methods produce figures that guide the changes and viability of health insurance plans, managed care, and health maintenance organizations (HMOs). Few physicians need to develop their own life tables, but many need to understand

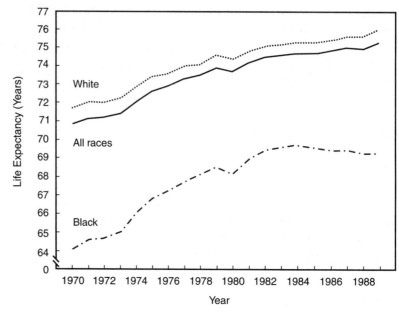

Figure 2-4.
Life expectancy at birth, by year of birth, and by race—United States, 1970 to 1989. (*MMWR* 1992;41:124.)

the basis of the figures (particularly those in columns 2 and 7 in Table 2-2) to ensure financial and organizational survival of the settings in which they work.

MORBIDITY

Reportable diseases are those that by law must be reported to health authorities. The list varies from state to state and from time to time according to the importance attributed to a given disease. Such reporting, if incomplete, gives a distorted picture of the frequency of disease in communities. Moreover, the incidence of many disease groups that do not usually kill people, such as mental illness and arthritis, is underrepresented in death rates. Attempts to require the reporting of noninfectious diseases have had some success, with cancer registries being the most common example.

The United States National Health Service (NHS) Health Survey is an attempt to correct these deficiencies of reporting through use of interviews of persons in a nationwide sample of households; other NHS surveys include use of medical examinations to provide clinical information that is not obtainable from interviews. These surveys provide good information on many nonfatal conditions in the US population.

Table 2-3 provides an example of national survey data from the National Health and Nutrition Examination Surveys (NHANES). These NHANES data provide not only prevalence data, but also information on trends in disease diagnosis and management. For ex-

TABLE 2-2.
Abridged Life Table, United States, 1981

Age Interval	Proportion Dying	Of 100,000 Born Alive		Stationary Population		Average Remaining Lifetime
Period of Life Between Two Exact Ages Stated in Years (1)	Proportion of Persons Alive at Beginning of Age Interval Dying During Interval (2)	Number Living at Beginning of Age Interval (3)	Number Dying During Age Interval (4)	In the Age Interval (5)	In This and All Subsequent Age Intervals (6)	Average Number of Years of Life Remaining at Beginning of Age Interval (7)
$x + x + n$	$_nq_x$	l_x	$_nd_x$	$_nL_x$	T_x	e_x
All races						
0–1	0.0119	100,000	1,194	98,965	7,417,771	74.2
1–5	0.0024	98,806	236	394,675	7,318,806	74.1
5–10	0.0015	98,570	144	492,463	6,924,131	70.2
10–15	0.0015	98,426	146	491,822	6,431,668	65.3
15–20	0.0045	98,280	447	490,386	5,939,846	60.4
20–25	0.0061	97,833	598	487,689	5,449,460	55.7
25–30	0.0064	97,235	624	484,615	4,961,771	51.0
30–35	0.0068	96,611	655	481,489	4,477,156	46.3
35–40	0.0090	95,956	859	477,770	3,995,667	41.6
40–45	0.0134	95,097	1,277	472,503	3,517,897	37.0
45–50	0.0219	93,820	2,053	464,288	3,045,394	32.5
50–55	0.0344	91,767	3,161	451,424	2,581,106	28.1
55–60	0.0521	88,606	4,617	432,110	2,129,682	24.0
60–65	0.0776	83,989	6,521	404,395	1,697,572	20.2
65–70	0.1141	77,468	8,837	366,109	1,293,177	16.7
70–75	0.1648	68,631	11,309	315,778	927,068	13.5
75–80	0.2335	57,322	13,386	253,613	611,290	10.7
80–85	0.3450	43,936	15,158	181,171	357,677	8.1
85 and older	1.000	28,778	28,778	176,506	176,506	6.1

TABLE 2-3.

Age-Adjusted Prevalence of Hypertension, Percentage of the Population Receiving Prescription Drug Therapy for Hypertension, and Crude Rates of Treatment for Hypertension by Quintile of Body Mass Index in NHANES II and III

	Age-Adjusted Prevalence		Population Treated		Hypertension Treated	
	NHANES II (1976–1980)	NHANES III Phase 1 (1988–1991)	NHANES II (1976–1980)	NHANES III Phase 1 (1988–1991)	NHANES II (1976–1980)	NHANES III Phase 1 (1988–1991)
Overall	32	20	10	11	31	55
BMI quintile						
Quintile 1	18	11	6	6	28	53
Quintile 2	25	13	7	5	30	35
Quintile 3	33	21	9	11	29	54
Quintile 4	45	23	13	13	32	59
Quintile 5	58	34	19	19	37	61

NHANES, National Health and Nutrition Examination Survey; BMI, body mass index. Values are percents. BMI quintile cutoffs (weight/height²) were calculated from NHANES III data.

ample, comparing NHANES I (1976 to 1980) to NHANES II, Phase I (1988 to 1991) suggests improvements in proportions of hypertensive patients undergoing treatment from the late 1970s as compared with the 1988 to 1991 NHANES II, Phase II data.

ADMINISTRATION OF HEALTH CARE SERVICES

Good administration of public health services should ensure that individuals needing health care will receive it promptly and effectively, using measures that are readily accepted and understood by consumers. The nature of public health programs has changed markedly over the years. The earliest efforts were to prevent the introduction and the spread of infection by quarantine of ships or infected communities and isolation of infectious cases. As knowledge grew concerning infectious disease, the control of water supplies, milk, and many other foods was found to be necessary. Control of the disposal of human, household, and industrial wastes also was found to improve the health of the people, as did improvements in housing conditions.

In some parts of the world, government became involved in control or eradication of disease carriers, such as certain species of insects. Particularly in the United States and Western Europe, social reforms have taken place in which public health has been an important issue. Governments have become greatly interested in maternal and child welfare, in aid to the physically handicapped, and in special problems concerning such diseases as tuberculosis, venereal disease, cancer, cardiovascular disease, and mental illness. Indeed, rehabilitation, the early detection of chronic illness, and the assurance of continuity of medical care are becoming touchstones of modern public health. The increasing cost and better distribution and financing of personal health services also became leading concerns of the US government in the 1990s.

Whereas the previous emphasis of public health administration was on the establishment of basic public health services, there has come to be equal emphasis placed on the better use of existing services and the development and evaluation of new programs. In theory, new developments in public health should reduce the need for individual action (such as regular visits to the dentist) and motivate larger numbers of individuals to participate in voluntary programs. These developments have changed materially the character of government organization for the protection of the public health. The impersonal mass approach through environmental controls is being complemented by the financing of personal health services and by controlling the increasing cost of health care.

FEDERAL HEALTH SERVICES

The political structure and beliefs in the United States have guided the historical development of its public health services. A national government formed by a federation of the member states possesses only those powers delegated to it by the sovereign states. Article I of the Constitution of the United States provides for the federal government interest in the general welfare and gave some basis in authority for the development of national health services. The Constitution also delegated power to the federal government specifically for interstate and foreign quarantine.

In 1980, Congress created the Department of Health and Human Services (HHS), combining some of the federal agencies involved in health care services and regulation. Many health activities remain in other departments of the national government, such as the Veterans Administration, which is involved in extensive health efforts, the Armed Forces, the Occupational Safety and Health Administration (OSHA), and the Environmental Protection Agency (EPA).

US Department of Health and Human Services

The Public Health Service is one of the principal federal agencies concerned with public health. Originally formed to provide health care to sailors in the merchant marine, its functions have come to include interstate and international quarantine, research and demonstration programs, advice on technical matters, and the loan of personnel to other agencies with health services. A significant impact on health services is made through financial support to state and local health agencies for the expansion and improvement of their programs.

Health Care Financing Administration

Established in 1977, the Health Care Financing Administration (HCFA) is the federal agency responsible for Medicaid and Medicare, both launched in 1966. It also guides the activities of peer review organizations (PROs), which monitor length of stay and quality of hospital care through peer review efforts. Medicaid and Medicare currently form more than two thirds of the total federal budget on health. Medicare is equally managed health insurance for the elderly set up by the Social Security Act for persons 65 years of age or older, or for individuals with social security from a disability. Part A provides coverage for hospital expenses and Part B for physician expenses. Medicaid is financial aid to the poor for medical expenses. Medicaid is a state and federal administered program and is funded out of general tax revenues.

STATE AND LOCAL HEALTH ORGANIZATIONS

The state government is the sovereign power in the United States. In theory, the national and local governments possess only those powers delegated to them by the states. In practice, however, financial strength has given the federal government more influence in the development of state and local health programs than might otherwise have occurred.

Health laws differ greatly among the 50 states. In some, there is extensive, detailed health legislation; in others, only broad principles are laid down, and special laws are enacted as urgent needs are recognized. All states make some provision for a board of health or a comparable body with advisory and legislative functions.

In most states, the state health officer is a physician appointed by the governor with the advice of the state board of health. The state health officer's qualifications, duties, and compensation are usually specified by law. In the early years of the state health departments, control of communicable disease was the first objective, followed by environmental sanitation, dealing with water supply, and the safe disposal of wastes. In recent years, some states have created environmental protection agencies that have taken over most environmental services. They correspond to the EPA and to the OSHA on the national level.

Other responsibilities of state health departments include supplying maternal and child health services, recording health statistics, ensuring medical and hospital care for special groups, and providing certain long-term care and rehabilitation services. Most state health departments have a division of local health services to provide grants-in-aid to local communities and to advise local health departments. Most local health services are maintained by cities or counties, whereas the state delegates authority and often provides funds to the local community for developing the program. Local health departments give direct services, such as water purification and the supervision of sewage disposal, and a wide range of clinical services. Sparsely populated areas have only limited public health services, and in a few states the state health department directly provides local health services to its residents.

VOLUNTARY HEALTH AGENCIES

A voluntary health agency is formed by a group of members who have a common interest; membership is voluntary, and the agency is independent of the state. Although the United States is reputed to be a nation of joiners, only about 20% of the US population participate actively in its 100,000 voluntary health agencies. Such associations have become more common as society has grown more complex and activities more numerous. In situations of rapid social change, voluntary associations are considered to be important as a means of achieving new goals, raising new funds, or providing new labor.

Ideally, the voluntary health agency is more sensitive than the government to the changing needs of society; many agencies have initiated health programs that were later assumed by government. In recent years, however, as many voluntary agencies have become more stable and conservative, government agencies have become increasingly innovative. As the vitality of voluntary health agencies has decreased, public resistance has risen against giving funds for health activities over and above the taxes paid to government. It is now accepted policy to have voluntary associations carry out public functions, such as payment for medical and hospital care and professional licensure; thus, some voluntary agencies, such as Blue Cross/Blue Shield, receive increasing support from government funds.

Voluntary health agencies take many forms:

1. A large group of agencies focus on specific diseases (e.g., American Cancer Society) or specific organs (e.g., American Heart Association), or on specific populations or techniques (e.g., Planned Parenthood). These agencies concentrate more on health education and less on service.

2. HMOs are medical groups that contract with an enrolled population to provide complete health services, preventive and curative, inpatient and outpatient, in return for an annual payment per enrollee.
3. Foundations, such as the Robert Wood Johnson or Kellogg foundations, distribute funds to nonprofit groups for service, research, and educational activities.
4. Planning and coordinating associations, such as community councils, form a fourth group of voluntary agencies.
5. Professional associations, such as the American Medical Association, are composed of influential groups concerned with setting standards for and licensing the profession, and with public and professional education and legislation related to the beliefs and activities of the profession. State and local medical societies also guide most PROs, even though federal funds support their reviews of hospital care.
6. Some academic institutions may be included that are concerned with the research and teaching of health professionals.

Voluntary health associations can stimulate social change and help focus on research priorities. They help communities set priorities in health and influence the decisions of local government. They create interest and consensus among their members but also induce stresses between one organization and another. If this conflict results in improved health services for a reasonable expenditure of funds, the results will be helpful to society. However, the way one views voluntarism must be based on intuition, social values, and personal opinion rather than on scientific findings, because, to date, no conclusive research exists to settle the question.

OCCUPATIONAL HEALTH

Occupational health is concerned with all factors that influence the health and productivity of working people. A wide variety of occupational hazards pose significant risks to health. Within the federal government, the National Institute for Occupational Safety and Health (NIOSH) estimates that 10 million persons are injured, 3 million severely, while at work each year. About 70,000 injuries result in permanent impairment. Of nontraumatic illness, skin diseases account for the highest proportion of occupational illness.

In recent years, hospitals and medical groups have begun to deliver occupational health programs to smaller industries. More physicians have become better trained in the diagnosis and treatment of occupational illness. These steps have been motivated as much by the need to improve revenue of delivery programs as by the need to improve occupational health in society.

Occupational health physicians and labor unions have been particularly active in prevention and treatment of diseases that arise either in the course of employment or as a result of work. Recently, however, employers have also become more interested in workplace-based health promotion programs. When health care costs became so large that they began to influence profits, employers became more interested in self-help and self-care programs for employees. Growth of the managed-care-for-profit health care sector, with its continuing need to contain costs, is also changing the way of providing health programs and facilities at the workplace.

Both governmental and private health programs at the work site tend to emphasize prevention and improved health, morale, and job satisfaction. These programs also promote safety and accident control, as well as reduce health risks such as smoking, hypertension, poor diet, alcohol abuse, and occupational related illness. When effective, these programs improve health and productivity and control health care costs. However, scientific studies are needed to document that the benefits of work site health promotion activities outweigh their costs.

Within the federal government, NIOSH conducts research and recommends standards for toxic substances used in industry; implementing that information, OSHA promulgates standards and inspects industries to ensure compliance.

TOXIC AGENTS AND RADIATION

For decades, concern has grown over the condition of the environment and its effect on health and quality of life. In 1970, the federal EPA was created and began to set national air, water, and other pollution standards. In 1976, the Toxic Substances Control Act identified the need to control the risk of exposure to **65,000 commercial chemicals, about which there is good information on health hazards for only 2%.** In 1980, a federal act known as Superfund recognized the need to clean up thousands of hazardous waste sites in the United States. To date, only a fraction of these sites have been cleaned up.

Low-level ionizing radiation occurs naturally and also comes from medical x-rays. Much higher doses of radiation are known to be carcinogenic, mutagenic, and teratogenic. Most Americans are exposed to 200 mrem or less of ionizing radiation per year. In the 1980s, a naturally occurring radioactive gas called *radon* was recognized as potentially dangerous to health.

The regulatory agencies EPA and OSHA historically have been understaffed for the enforcement of the many laws that control the use and disposal of hazardous substances in the environment. Ideally, new chemicals should be withheld from use until industry can demonstrate safety. Unfortunately, epidemiologic studies of human populations can demonstrate harm, but they rarely arrive at precise dose-response relationships. The permissible exposure levels must reflect real-life multiple exposures, the history of previous exposure, individual susceptibilities, and the changing effects with increasing age. Safety standards must, therefore, be negotiated between interest groups.

Pharmaceutical and biologic hazards also deserve full attention. We have yet to resolve the conflicting social goals of increased consumption, industrial expansion, and adequate health protection in the United States. Because the balance is complex, one should not depend on mechanistic decision making using simple cost-benefit analysis. Unfortunately, the political stresses involved in the public environment debates discourage all but the most insensitive and the most dedicated professionals from becoming involved.

ACCIDENT PREVENTION AND INJURY CONTROL

In the United States, accidents rank fourth as a cause of death; they lead in causing death up to the age of 44 years. **Motor vehicle accidents cause about half of all accidental deaths.** Among the elderly, in whom accidents cause a proportionately lower incidence of death and disability, the combination of osteoporosis with falls has raised interest in the prevention of hip fractures.

Among those dying in motor vehicle accidents, about half involve the use of alcohol by one or both the drivers. Accident patients receiving treatment in hospital emergency departments also include significant numbers with alcohol detected in their blood, including more than half of those injured in fights or assaults. All accidents do not result in death. Injury without death is one of the leading causes of visits to physicians' offices. Personal and social problems are common among accident repeaters. Thus, it is obviously clear that the host factors such as alcohol abuse are important in determining the incidence of accidents.

Technologic changes such as improved automobile design (e.g., air bags) and passive measures such as window guards for apartment buildings have been very effective in preventing injuries. Regulatory measures such as building codes, fire codes, reduced highway speed limits, and the reduced availability of handguns through licensing have also been effective. Economic incentives are also a potentially strong source of improved prevention. These incentives include low insurance rates for documented safe drivers, higher taxes on cigarettes and alcohol, and lower life insurance rates for those who use no alcohol or cigarettes. The field of injury control, therefore, involves multiple measures. Physicians can help by using their social stature as role models and by their counseling.

DENTAL HEALTH

Periodic surveys of dental health problems indicate that the nation's dental health has improved in recent decades in the United States. The prospects for further prevention of dental problems continue to be encouraging. The use of fluoride at optimal levels before and after the eruption of permanent teeth has reduced the amount of dental caries by more than one half.

Dental caries in the past was a massive health problem. Even in the 1990s, low-income children have many more untreated decayed teeth than high-income children. Fluoride, which is in the water supply for the majority of the United States population, delays the onset of dental caries and reduces the need for treatment by dentists. Prepayment for dental care through dental insurance has become a job-related benefit of many employees.

Half of all caries develop in the pits and grooves of the chewing surfaces of teeth, where the fluoride seems to be least effective. Dental sealants are plastic resins that are applied to these surfaces to prevent further decay. These sealants appear to be very effective, but dentists have been slow to use them, possibly because of unfamiliarity as well as concerns about future economic consequences.

ECONOMICS OF HEALTH CARE

If current health behavior were understood, one would become more effective in persuading people to improve this behavior. One might expect that the use of health services depends primarily on the frequency of disease or discomfort suffered by individuals or groups. This expectation, however, is only partly true. For the many preventable or treatable conditions that are more common in lower income groups, persons at greatest risk use health care and take preventive measures less often than those at lower risk.

Compared with higher income groups, the poor have higher infant mortality rates, a higher incidence of infectious disease, higher incidence of hypertension, a higher incidence of end-stage renal disease, and a higher prevalence of untreated dental disease. However, almost all surveys show that the poor have lower utilization rates of preventive and ambulatory health care. Within each poverty level, African Americans usually show lower utilization rates than whites.

Hospital admission rates are high, both for the poor and non-poor, but the former have longer duration of stay. Such findings suggest that the poor delay longer before seeking care, and when they are admitted, more serious illness has developed. This interpretation is confirmed by the finding that for almost every diagnostic group, death is a more frequent outcome among the lower income patients admitted to hospital.

Health care has a number of characteristics that distinguish it from other types of services and commodities. First, health care may produce external benefits; thus, health care includes many procedures that benefit society as well as the individual who receives the service. Second, besides being a consumption commodity—something that is used up and money is spent on—health care is partly a good investment; dollars spent on health care may raise future productivity and return the same dollars with interest. Third, certain health services have a collective value when used by one person, and there is no decrease in availability to others. For example, when one person consumes fluoridated water, an abundance remains to give the benefits of fluoridation to other drinkers. The large dollar investment needed—such as for water and sewer systems, or for the buildings and personnel to provide hospital or nursing home care— also applies to many health services.

The amount in dollars that individuals are willing to pay for preventive measures tends to be below the true value to society; generally, the individual does not care to pay for the additional benefits to society or for intangible future benefits. When the income of the average American family doubles, its demand for preventive care more than doubles, whereas that for curative care increases less. However, low-income families give priority to treatment when ill, and they regard as less urgent and relevant preventive measures that are also indicated for continued good health. Thus, a strong argument can be made that government funds should support a number of health services and should, in particular, be funneled into preventive health services. The political controversy over the appropriate area for government funds has primarily supported curative care. Science does not guide the development of a consensus on this point, and future decisions will arise politically.

In recent years the costs of medical care have risen more steeply than other costs in the United States, particularly in the field of hospital care. The main reasons for the increase in hospital costs have been the following:

1. In previous years, hospitals required many employees to work long hours at low wages. Since the 1960s, the gap in wages and working conditions between hospitals and other industries has gotten smaller.
2. Technical and scientific advances have increased the complexity of hospital care. Rarely does an improvement replace a step that was more expensive; most often, the innovation forms an extra step intended to improve the quality of care.
3. Hospitals make intensive use of human services; they have not raised their productivity as fast as has the economy at large.
4. Some educational and training programs cost more than the value of the benefits obtained. Part of inpatient hospital charges finances the training of nurses and physicians.
5. With insurance and subsidies, consumers face a price for health

care that is below the true cost of providing it, causing consumers to purchase more than they otherwise would.

An increasing amount of money spent on health services comes from health insurance plans, sometimes described as third party payments. Persons with hospital insurance have higher rates of inpatient hospital use than those without insurance. However, the evidence suggests that those without insurance have greater, rather than less, need for hospitalization. The government-financed Medicare program helped reduce this problem for persons aged 65 years or older but does not eliminate it. The debate on nationwide compulsory health insurance focuses on the need for better coverage of other groups as well. In 1998, 16% of Americans did not have health insurance.

With third party payments, increasing prices cause less individual protest and less change in use than when the individual pays directly for care. Thus, the price of a health service does not relate so inversely to its consumption as does price in other fields. Other rationing devices tend to develop when the price mechanism is not effective. Waiting lists for services develop, and registration at outpatient clinics may become unpleasant, partly to discourage a rapid return of patients. These deterrents have a different impact on different groups; price deters high-income patients less than low-income ones; long waiting times deter the unemployed less than those eager to return to the job they hold.

Federal legislation in 1982 detailed a payment-per-case system for general hospital care of Medicare inpatients. Each patient is placed into 1 of 470 mutually exclusive classes called *diagnosis-related groups* (DRGs). Based partly on the principal diagnosis, complications, and treatment procedures used, the assigned DRG leads to the "appropriate" payment for care, which is unchanged whether the stay is short or long. Intended to control costs without weakening quality, the actual effect of widely using DRGs has been to discharge patients more quickly at a more seriously ill stage.

HEALTH CARE FACILITIES

The system of health care facilities can be pictured as forming a bridge that carries the individual seeking help to the health worker who provides that service. The system also provides the necessary equipment and technology to make the service as effective as possible.

There is no ideal system of health care. The way in which personal health services and facilities are organized depends mainly on factors outside the control of health professionals. The most prominent characteristics of the existing system of health care facilities are its complexity and the difficulty it has in responding to the conflicting demands of quality versus cost.

Although there is no ideal pattern of organization, the goals to be aimed at are clearer than they were in the past. Health care services ideally should be organized so that they are

1. Readily accessible, with no socioeconomic or geographic barriers that discriminate among population groups
2. Adequate in quantity, providing enough of each necessary service
3. Comprehensive, covering the range of needed services and facilitating continuity of care
4. Effective, reaching their stated goals, which will become more ambitious as techniques improve
5. Efficient, reaching their goals with a reasonable degree of economy
6. Of good quality, satisfying the consumer as well as the producer of health services

As of 1998, the US health care system has failed to achieve these goals. It remains to be seen whether the massive US experiment in managed care will perform better. More systematic coordination of health care services and monitoring quality are critical needs.

Hospitals

In the forefront of the US health care facilities is the acute general hospital, whose orientation has always been toward the treatment of existing diseases. At times, its policy makers have paid lip service to health promotion and disease prevention, but rarely have these activities been regarded as higher than public relations efforts. In recent years, general hospitals have found their financial viability in danger, and efforts have been made to consolidate and broaden the hospital activities. Hospital survival relates most strongly to providing quality care, with a reasonable amount of efficiency. Such cost-control efforts as the DRGs in Medicare, as well as managed care, have raised the cost of each patient-day but have also speeded the discharge of patients so that total cost per stay is lower.

Personnel

Since 1970, the number of people employed in health care has more than doubled. In that period, physician population ratios have increased about 40%, without much improvement in the regional variation in the supply of physicians. Thus, physicians continue to be most abundant in the Northeast and are most scarce in the South. Community hospitals continue to be the largest employers of personnel in health care.

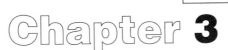

Chapter 3

Medical Statistics

To most medical students and house staff, the word *statistics* conventionally conjures up all kinds of negative images. Statistics seems to be a discipline that is far removed from the diagnosis and treatment of illness. Most physicians were exposed in the first year or two of medical school to an obligatory statistics or public health course provided in one of a variety of formats in some of the least appreciated of all medical school courses. The material seemed remote from patient care, the "real" mission of medical school. Later, during residency, is when biostatistics can be appreciated, when clinicians find themselves late at night in the hospital library, desperately trying to interpret the relevant studies that deal with critically important clinical decisions about treatment. This chapter presents basic concepts of medical statistics that all physicians should be familiar with.

Physicians who care for patients are constantly stating hypotheses and forming opinions on diagnosis and treatments based at least in part on clinical experience. Relying only on clinical experience to make such decisions is hazardous because of its inevitable bias and random associations. Clinical research is essential to guiding treatment decisions, and medical statistics is the primary tool for separating what is real from random variation.

BIOLOGIC VARIABILITY

To understand statistics it is necessary to understand biologic variability. Biologic measures (variables) in medicine are not set at specific levels; rather, they are changing constantly, moving up or down around an average or mean. This is true of blood pressure, pulse, temperature, white blood cell count—in fact, every biologic measure, even height, changes over time. The distance in which this movement occurs is measurable and predictable according to the standard deviation (SD). Understanding and managing this **inherent variability of biologic measures is the crux of biostatistics.**

NORMAL DISTRIBUTION

Essentially, all biologic measures are in a state of constant change. The variations can be described and interpreted, and most biologic variables are usually **normally distributed** (also called **Gaussian distribution**).

Understanding characteristics of the normal distribution is needed to understand biostatistics. Important concepts for this understanding include: **mean (x),** which is the average or the sum of all individual measurements divided by the total numbers of measurements; **SD (σ),** a measure of degree of variability or dispersion of the measure. The mean and SD can be expressed in terms of populations or samples. Figure 3-1 illustrates a normal distribution. As can be seen in this figure, a normal distribution ± 2 SD encompasses 95% of the measures and ± 3 SD encompasses 99.7%. In addition to the mean, there are two additional ways to describe central tendency of data: the mode and the median. The **mode** is defined as the most frequent single value found in the data. For example, the most common systolic blood pressure in a normal distribution is 126 mmHg. The **median** is the middle value of the data ranked from lowest to the highest. In a distribution, half of the values are to the left of the median, the other half to the right. The mode and median are often used when analyzing small data sets in which the mean value does not describe the central tendency well. Figure 3-2 illustrates the mean, median, and mode in a sample distribution.

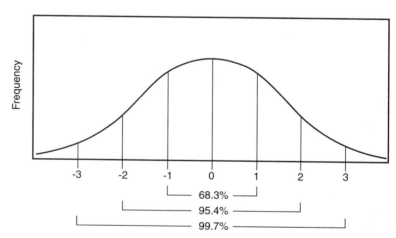

Figure 3-1.
Normal distribution curve.

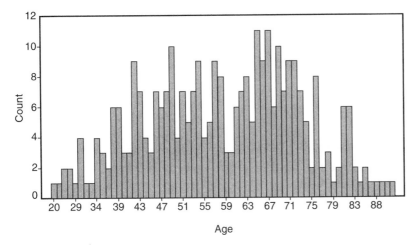

Mean: 58.6 yrs.   Median: 59 yrs.   Mode: 65 and 67 yrs. (bimodal distribution)

Figure 3-2.
Age distribution of 307 medical patients.

MEASURES OF VARIABILITY

The SD and standard error (SE) are two measures of variability that are widely used in reporting results from medical studies. SD (σ) is derived from the measure called **variance** (σ^2), which is the average squared deviation about the mean: $\Sigma (x - u)^2$. The SD is the square root of the variance. Another useful measure is the **coefficient of variation (CV),** which is the SD divided by the mean, or CV = σ/x. CV is commonly used to assess the reliability of medical tests (e.g., serum cholesterol). The **SE** is used to describe the distribution of a sample statistic and is derived from the SD and the sample size: $SE_x = \sigma/\sqrt{n}$. SE is frequently used in analyzing studies that compare the extent of differences between two different sample means.

COMMON STATISTICAL TESTS

Some of the commonly used statistical tests follow.

Student's t Test

The student's t test is a commonly used test for comparing mean values of two different groups. This test is used with continuous variables and provides the ability to estimate what the likelihood of differences in means are or are not (as a result of chance variations).

Student t tests are further described as unpaired and paired: **unpaired t tests** for differences in two treatment groups in which different patients are compared and **paired t tests** for comparisons before and after treatments given in the same subject.

Analysis of Variance

Analysis of variance (**ANOVA**) is used to analyze for result differences among several treatment groups. Here the **"F statistic"** is used to estimate probabilities that treatment groups are different.

$$F = \frac{\text{group variance estimated from sample means}}{\text{group variance estimated as average of sample variances}}$$

Multivariate Analysis

Multivariate analysis is a statistical means to examine the relationship among many factors (variables) considered together.

Wilcoxon Signed Ranks Test

Wilcoxon signed ranks test is a nonparametric test that compares two dependent samples with ordinal data or continuous variables that are not normally distributed.

Mantel-Haenzel Chi-Square Test

The Mantel-Haenzel chi-square test is a test of two or more 2×2 contingency tables designed to test for differences in proportions.

Fisher's Exact Test

Fisher's exact test is used with 2×2 contingency tables when chi-square tests cannot be done because of small sample size.

P VALUES

Quantitative research using clinical measures by necessity involves statistical testing. The likelihood that a treatment is different from control (better or worse) is expressed as a **"P value,"** or probability value. Traditionally, P values are considered **statistically significant** if they are less than or equal to 0.05; in other words, if identical studies were repeated 100 times, the particular result would be expected to occur in only 5% or fewer of the studies as a result of chance alone. So P values measure the extent of dissimilarity between results of different groups.

The convention of P values of less than or equal to 0.05 being "significant" is arbitrary; a P value of 0.07, although not reaching the <0.05 level, means that in 100 repetitions of the same study, one would expect that result by chance in only 7 of 100 outcomes. For a P value of 0.10, the result by chance would be 1 in 10, for a P value of 0.20, the result would be one in five, and for 0.50, the observed difference is "50/50."

The smaller the P value, the stronger is the likelihood that the observed difference is real, that is, not due to chance. For example, a P value of <0.01 = less than 1 in 100 chance, 0.001 = only 1 in 1000 chance, and so on.

It is preferable to give the actual P value in literature rather than simply stating "significant" or "nonsignificant," because the actual value conveys much more information. The actual P value also depends on whether the statistical test is one tailed (one sided) or two tailed (two sided). With a one-sided test, the direction of the hypothesis is one way; for example, the hypothesis is "the treatment is better than placebo." A two-tailed test allows for the possibility that the treatment could be beneficial or harmful compared to control. Two-tailed testing is much more conservative and is almost always the test of choice.

It is important not to equate statistical significance to clinical importance. If the study sample is large enough (which is rarely the case), then minor differences can be statistically significant but not clinically relevant.

CONFOUNDING AND BIAS

Confounding and bias are two of the most important concepts for understanding in interpreting and evaluating the medical literature. Not understanding these concepts can sometimes lead to dangerous misinterpretations.

Confounding

Confounding is when two variables are closely associated with one another so that one obscures or confuses the true relationship to a third variable.

Example 1: Early studies observed a strong positive relationship between level of sugar intake and incidence of coronary heart disease

(CHD). However, sugar in the diet is also closely tied to dietary *fat*, after controlling for sugar intake, it was clear that the *true* independent relationship was with fat and CHD. In this case, the relationship of sugar and CHD was confounded by fat intake.

Example 2: In several observational cross-sectional studies, it has been observed that cigarette smokers have lower levels of blood pressure compared to nonsmokers. Based on these observations, it has been suggested that cigarette smoking may cause blood pressure to decline. However, this relationship appears because smokers systematically weigh less than nonsmokers. Body weight is strongly and positively related to blood pressure. The true relationship of blood pressure to smoking is confounded by body weight. Other common confounders are age, alcohol intake, and treatment selection.

One method used to determine whether confounding is operating is to *adjust* the data so that the data are independent of the potentially confounding variables. For example, smoking-adjusted rates would take into account smoking levels in the population and would show that smoking and blood pressure are not related once the relationship of smoking to body mass index has been taken into account.

Bias

Bias is similar to confounding. Bias is the process that tends to produce results that differ from the true results. Frequently, bias is related to how study groups differ. All forms of bias threaten the validity of an observation or study. There are several different forms of bias and the following discussion gives examples of the more common ones encountered in medical studies.

Measurement Bias

Measurement bias can be divided into two general areas: observer bias and technical bias. **Observer bias** occurs when the individual who does the measurement is biased. For example, this bias is seen in the terminal digit preference method of measuring blood pressure. Most official guidelines for blood pressure measurement recommend rounding up blood pressure measures to the nearest even number (e.g., systolic 140, 142, 144 mm Hg). Given this guideline, there are only five possible terminal digits: 0, 2, 4, 6, and 8. In a pressure of 138/90, the 8 is the systolic terminal digit and the 0 is the diastolic terminal digit. Because there are five possible terminal digits, in a variable with a normal distribution and a large number of measures, each terminal digit should be represented in about 20% of the measures. However, when actual data sets are examined, certain terminal digits are preferred by the observer. Table 3-1 shows terminal digit data from the large Hypertension Detection and Follow-up Program's community screening. Zero makes up the largest percentage and 4 makes up the least. These observational preferences can be very strong. In fact, past studies have found that the most prevalent

TABLE 3-1.

Blood Pressure Terminal Digit Preference at the Initial Screen for Eligibility into the Hypertension Detection and Follow-up Program (HDFP)

Systolic Blood Pressure Terminal Digit	Blood Pressure Measures (n)	Percent
0	63,315	40.0
2	24,695	15.6
4	22,708	14.3
6	20,044	12.7
8	27,501	17.4

overall blood pressure value when *physicians* measure blood pressure (the mode) is 120/80 mm Hg, a measure commonly considered "normal" blood pressure. Physicians have a strong preference for 0 as the terminal digit.

Technical bias reflects the measurement process itself and usually involves differences in the equipment (e.g., mercury manometers that are poorly maintained) or the environment (e.g., failure to standardize the measurement procedure). Technical bias can also be a problem in biochemical measures; for example, measurements made with a new analyzer in a laboratory frequently vary significantly from those made with an existing one.

Selection Bias

In the literature, **selection bias is one of the most common forms of bias** encountered. For example, data from a large blood pressure control trial that used thiazide diuretics and reserpine showed that hypertensive patients in the study were 50% *less* likely to report depression on reserpine compared to thiazide. This was a surprising result because reserpine was widely believed to cause depression. This odd result could be explained by selection bias. Patients who had a history of depression or who appeared depressed were initially given the diuretic selectively and reserpine was avoided.

Endpoint Ascertainment Bias

This bias occurs when study groups have different opportunities or chances to have their disease or endpoint detected. For example, in a study in which the treatment group is being seen in the clinic every 3 months and the control group is seen once a year, then members of the treatment group have many more opportunities to report on study events, such as illnesses and hospitalizations. Also, the group with more frequent visits would know the staff better, feel more comfortable in the clinic, and be more willing or even eager to report on symptoms. Endpoint ascertainment bias can be a major threat to the integrity of a study. The best way to minimize this bias is to standardize the frequency of contact and make sure that the observers assigning the study endpoints are not aware of, or are blinded to, the patient study group. Endpoint ascertainment bias can also occur when the study investigators who see trial patients are also involved in defining the endpoint (e.g., the endpoint is defined as myocardial infarction). This form of bias is particularly a problem in open treatment (unblinded) studies in which physicians may have strong preferences for certain drugs used in the study.

Treatment Selection Bias

Treatment selection bias is a common source of bias that can be observed in a variety of study types and can lead to serious errors in interpreting results. Treatment selection bias also is frequently an issue in case-control studies. For example, one case-control study observed that hypertensive patients receiving calcium channel blocking drugs were 60% *more* likely to experience a fatal or nonfatal myocardial infarction compared to patients given standard drugs (mostly diuretics and beta blockers) (Table 3-2). It was suggested from these study results that calcium channel blockers may be "causing" myocardial infarctions. It is also likely, however, that physicians are more likely to give calcium channel blockers to patients who are at higher risk for

TABLE 3-2.

Case-Control Study Examining the Association Between Myocardial Infarction and Antihypertensive Derived from a Large Managed Care Data Set

Drug	Cases (n)	Controls (n)	Adjusted RR (95% CI)
Diuretics			
Alone	99	452	1.0 (reference)
Beta blockers			
Alone	51	234	1.09 (0.74–1.63)
With diuretics	34	161	0.97 (0.62–1.52)
Calcium channel blockers			
Alone	56	170	1.58 (1.04–2.39)
With diuretics	24	60	1.70 (0.97–2.99)
ACE inhibitors			
Alone	32	159	1.01 (0.62–1.62)
With diuretics	10	66	0.66 (0.32–1.37)
Vasodilators			
Alone	16	43	1.53 (0.79–2.97)
With diuretics	13	50	0.91 (0.46–1.83)

ACE, angiotensin-converting enzyme.

development of the disease. (Calcium channel blockers are used to treat angina pectoralis.) If this was the case, then calcium channel blockers would be a surrogate for higher risk of development of the disease. This "chicken-egg" dilemma is an inherent problem in all case-control studies. Case-control studies cannot establish causation but these studies do raise important questions that can then establish causation through clinical trials.

Design Bias

Study designs from the outset can be faulty and result in bias. For example, in one hypertension treatment trial comparing two different agents, if blood pressure was uncontrolled or the assigned drug stopped, then the protocol called for starting the other study drug. At the end of the study, the proportion of patients on drug A and on drug B were almost identical. Without a treatment difference between study groups, the result was biased toward seeing "no difference."

Treatment Assignment Bias

Treatment assignment bias occurs when the study group or treatment assignment becomes to any degree predictable. For example, one study compared treatment of pneumococcal pneumonia with antibiotics, either penicillin or lincomycin. Treatment assignment was not randomized but carried out on an alternate day basis. Lobar pneumonia patients seen in the emergency department on Monday, Wednesday, and Friday were given penicillin; patients seen on Tuesday, Thursday, and Friday were given lincomycin.

In the emergency department, a patient's entry to the study was determined by the internal medicine resident. When the study was completed, the results showed no difference in death or complications between the antibiotics; in fact, there was a nonsignificant trend favoring lincomycin. This surprising result came about from treatment assignment bias. It was later discovered that severely ill pneumonia patients were intentionally not entered into the study or occasionally were even encouraged to return to the emergency department the next day. Why? Because the residents believed strongly that penicillin was the preferred treatment. This bias selectively placed more severe cases into the penicillin group. This example points out why randomization is crucial for treatment trials because it ensures that the **assignment is unpredictable.**

Study Dropout Bias

Study dropout bias is common. Study dropouts are participants who are voluntarily lost to follow-up. Patients who are dropouts are surely different from the participating patients. They tend to have different demographics, lifestyles, and number of study events. Dropout bias is much more problematic if the rate of dropouts is differential across study groups.

TESTING HYPOTHESES

Stating a hypothesis is a crucial first step in beginning a scientific investigation. A hypothesis can be stated in the null form (**null hypothesis**), which states that the treatment is the same as a placebo, or in an alternate form (**alternate hypothesis**), which states that a new treatment is better or worse than a placebo or an established therapy. Clearly stating the hypothesis to be tested is an important step, which later determines the study design and approaches to analyses, as well as the conclusions.

Two types of errors can be made in testing the hypothesis. One error occurs when a significant difference between treatments (**false positive**) is observed, but when, in reality, a true difference does not exist. This is called a **type I,** or **alpha** (α) **error.** Type I errors may be due to study bias or to chance from random variation. To help ensure that this error does not occur, the alpha level is set appropriately during the design phase of the study. Conventionally, alphas are set at 0.05, which means that, with the size sample in the study group, one would expect to see a significant difference by chance in only 1 of 20 similar experiments (5%). This alpha value corresponds to the "P values" considered statistically significant (usually at a P less than or equal to 0.05 value). This means that the difference between treatments is accepted as statistically significant only when the chance of a false-positive result is very low (<5%).

Although much less recognized or appreciated, the **type II error** is also critically important. A type II error is the error of concluding that two treatments are the same when, in reality, a true difference does in fact exist (**false negative**). Type II errors are also called **beta** (β) **errors.** When designing a study, beta errors are conventionally set somewhere between 0.95 and 0.80, meaning that when the study outcome shows no difference using a beta of 0.9, then 90% of the time when no difference is observed this result truly indicates no difference.

The **power** of a study is related most to the type II error; power is the likelihood that no type II error exists. The power of a study is highly dependent on the sample size of study; the larger the sample size, the greater the power. Power is also related to the precision with which the crucial variable can be studied and to the size of the treatment effect. The larger the treatment effect and the more precise (less variable) the measures, the greater the power. There are many small studies that conclude no effect of certain treatments but that have little power and so are likely to have made a type II error. Larger studies carried out later frequently show a significant effect of that treatment. Insufficient power is a major problem in clinical studies. However, specific statistical tests have been developed that examine whether treatments are different, and tests are available to compare differences in average or mean change and for categorical variables.

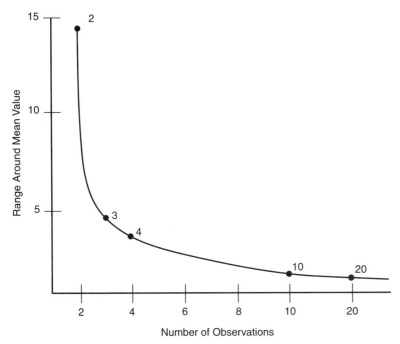

Figure 3-3.
Effect of repeated observations on precision of measurement.

Regression to the Mean

All biologic measures are in a state of constant flux, moving up or down around an average value. Measures such as height vary little and require measurement less often than measures that vary more often. Individual patients experience this variability, as do study groups and even populations. How variability influences inferences in study results has already been discussed. Variability also influences how one interprets individual patient responses. An important statistical and clinical phenomenon that results from this pattern of variability is called *regression to the mean*. **Regression to the mean** is defined as the tendency for measures that are initially obtained from persons selected using cutpoints that are set above or below the mean of the group to become more like the group mean on subsequent measures. For example, in a diabetic group with fasting glucose greater than or equal to 140 mg/dl selected from a group or population with a mean or average blood glucose of 90 mg/dl, repeat measurement will show *lower* values of glucose compared to the first measurement. These measurements will have *regressed toward the group mean*. This phenomenon, which may at first seem like an esoteric statistical concept, has great practical clinical significance as well as significance for interpreting the results of studies. Frequently, apparently favorable changes in studies that are credited to specific treatments or the "placebo effect" are really due to regression to the mean. Clinically, the concept is also useful. For example, it may help explain the phenomenon of "white coat hypertension," which is the observation that blood pressure measurement in some hypertensive patients is higher in the physician's office. Regression to the mean often can explain the tendency for abnormal laboratory values to be normal on repeat measurements.

Regression to the mean can be minimized or eliminated by standardizing the measurement process and by doing multiple measures over time and averaging those measures to arrive at the values used for purposes of record, either clinical management or scientific study. Figure 3-3 shows the relation of repeated measures of cholesterol and the tendency for regression to the mean as well as how the approximate additional measures are better than the true value. It is an important concept to be aware of because it will always operate if cutpoints are set, as they commonly are in clinical management and clinical studies.

Chapter 4

Epidemiology

Epidemiology may be the most important public health field related to community medicine; it also represents its closest link to clinical medicine. It is the "basic science" of community medicine. Epidemiology is the study of disease as it manifests itself in a *population*. As the word *epidemiology* implies, it has its roots in the study of infectious disease epidemics and efforts to understand the causes and means to prevent them. Epidemiology is characterized by the population perspective and rates of disease occurrence in the population. Whereas the focus of clinical medicine is on the individual cases, **epidemiology is concerned with the disease as well as the persons in the population who do not get the disease.** In comparing biologic, genetic, and environmental characteristics between cases and noncases, risk factors can be identified and hypotheses formulated about causation. Once causes are identified, prevention becomes a possibility. The ability to prevent disease can then be tested experimentally by using clinical trial methodology.

Some basic epidemiologic concepts originate from the field of infectious diseases. They suggest that the frequency of many diseases may be explained on the basis of a host (the susceptible person) interacting with an agent (the factor causing the disease) and with the environment (including its psychosocial, biologic, and other aspects). Also from the infectious disease field comes the concept of an **incubation (or latency) period,** that is, the time between exposure to a causal agent and the onset of disease. A third concept is that of **herd immunity;** this concept emphasizes the notion that populations will stop spreading infectious disease even before they are fully immunized against the condition. For example, in a population in which 70% of persons are immune to an infection, the person-to-person spread may never become established because the infectious agent reaches many individuals who do not transmit the disease. The proportion of the population that produces herd immunity varies with the infectivity of the agent and with the size and social behavior characteristics of the community. The phenomenon of herd immunity makes it unnecessary to have 100% participation in some immunization programs; it is customary, however, to aim at as close to that level as possible.

Epidemiologic concepts and methods can be applied to accidents, poisonings, measurements, attitudes, and, indeed, to any observable characteristic of people. Epidemiologic studies ideally involve all cases with a given characteristic or disease in a defined population, and information is collected on the unaffected as well as affected persons. Such studies often develop rates (or ratios) in which the numerator represents those with the characteristic under study, and the denominator represents the total population, both the affected and unaffected.

Besides the infectious diseases, contemporary epidemiology concerns itself with chronic diseases, especially cardiovascular diseases, cancer, and acquired immunodeficiency syndrome (AIDS), because these are the epidemics of modern times. Clinical epidemiology is a relatively new field, which is closely tied to academic clinical medicine. This field applies epidemiologic design and methods to clinical research questions and problems.

The primary methods of epidemiologic research include observational studies, case-control studies, clinical trials, and meta-analysis.

Observational Studies

Usually these are large prospective studies in which many measures or exposures are carried out at a point in time in a defined population, and then the population is systematically followed up at regular intervals for years or decades. In the observational study, there is no attempt made to intervene or change any factors. Follow-up involves reassessment of the measures of interest and ascertainment of the individuals in the population in whom the disease develops. Prevalence and incidence rates can be calculated for specific diseases, and risk of becoming *a case* based on baseline exposure is examined. An example of a classic observational study is the Framingham Heart Study, which began in 1949 and involved measuring numerous factors (e.g., blood pressure, blood cholesterol, cigarette smoking) in 5200 residents of this Massachusetts community. Participants have been followed up every 2 years for 50 years. This study and numerous similar studies have contributed much to what is currently known about cardiovascular risk factors. For example, heart disease was found to be three times more likely to develop in persons with serum cholesterol levels in the upper quintile or 20th percentile of the population (or in their ensuing years) than in persons with cholesterol levels in the lowest quintile. An example of observational study data formatted for risk by serum cholesterol level is shown in Figure 4-1. Observational studies have contributed greatly to understanding of disease occurrence and causation in the cardiovascular field as well as in other fields, such as cancer and infectious disease.

Case-Control Studies

The case-control study is another method useful in epidemiology for exploring differences between persons who get a disease and those who do not. Unlike the observational study, case-control studies identify people who already have a disease, for example, lung cancer.

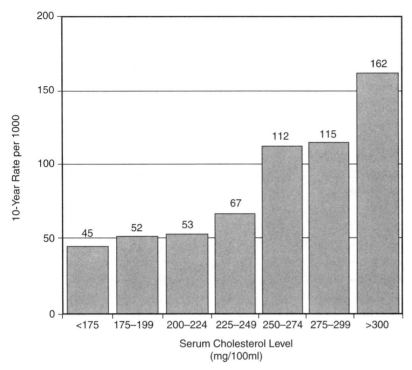

Figure 4-1.
Relationship of serum cholesterol and first coronary event in men 30 to 59 years old. (Data on serum cholesterol and risk from several observational studies—The Pooling Project.) (Blackburn H. *The American Heart Association Heartbook, A Guide to Prevention and Treatment of Cardiovascular Diseases,* p. 5. Dallas, The American Heart Association, 1980. Reproduced with permission. © Heartbook, A Guide to Prevention and Treatment of Cardiovascular Diseases, 1980. Copyright American Heart Association.)

Case-control studies are especially useful with diseases that are rare because recruiting enough persons with rare diseases is prohibitively expensive and logistically impossible. Identification of cases is often done from hospital admission records or disease registries. Potential exposures such as cigarette exposure, alcohol intake, and so forth are then catalogued. The cases are matched to control groups, usually for age, gender, and sometimes other important factors, such as education or income. Exposures are also ascertained in control groups. The groups are then compared to determine what exposures are different in control groups compared to cases. For example, cases of lung cancer have a higher rate of cigarette exposure than control groups. The ratio of the exposures in cases to control groups is called the **odds ratio.** For example, if smoking is 10 times more prevalent in lung cancer cases compared to control groups, then the odds ratio is 10. Case-control studies are useful in generating hypotheses about factors that cause a disease; however, they cannot prove causation because the timing of the exposure is usually not known. Also, it is difficult in case-control studies to identify proper control groups. Control groups selected from the community are generally more useful than those from hospitals.

Clinical Trials

The most sophisticated of epidemiologic methods is the clinical trial. In the clinical trial, the risk factor is actively changed or manipulated in one group. This factor is left unchanged or standard care is given in the comparison or control group. The disease incidence in both groups is tracked over time, and if the study is positive, a reduction in disease incidence compared to control subjects is observed in the treated group. The clinical trial is the best method of investigation for establishing causation. Clinical trials, however, are time-consuming and expensive, so they are generally only carried out with common conditions that have important medical, social, or economic consequences.

Clinical trials are frequently done using a procedure called blinding or masking. The main function of this procedure is to minimize bias. In a double-blind trial neither the participant nor the physician/ clinic staff are aware of the treatment assignment. Double-blind trials are frequently carried out with placebo controls. A single-blind trial is one in which either the participant or the physician/staff are aware of the treatment assigment but not both. Occasionally trials are referred to as triple-blind. Triple-blind means that not only is the participant and physician blinded to treatment assignment but the data monitoring committee examines the results unaware of treatment assignment. The study group looks at the results but the treatments are not specifically identified.

It is important that clinical trial results be analyzed according to intention to treat principles. Intention to treat means the final analysis includes all the participants randomized regardless of adherence to treatment or follow-up status.

Meta-analysis

Availability of resources and size of samples often limit the ability of any individual observational study or clinical trial to definitively answer the question posed. Conclusive studies, those in which there is a high level of confidence, generally require very large sample sizes and are, therefore, very expensive. Smaller studies have less statistical power, and frequently the outcomes of such studies indicate no evidence for benefit (or harm) when a larger study would have shown a difference (type II error).

Meta-analysis examines scientific questions by pooling results of similar studies to create a data set much larger than any individual study. With meta-analysis, the studies are the unit of analysis. For each separate study, the number of persons in the intervention group in whom disease developed are termed the *observed* events and they are contrasted with the *expected* events, assuming treatment does nothing. Calculation of the expected outcome, therefore, is based on the combined events, that is, disease in the intervention groups and disease in the control groups. If the intervention and treatment groups are no different, then the observed rate minus the expected rate would

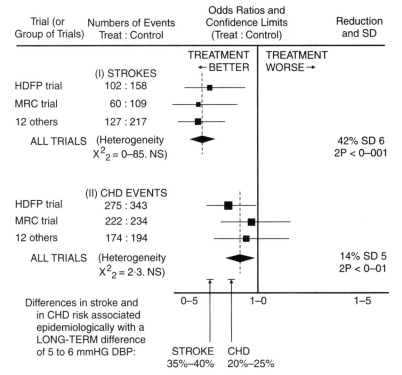

Figure 4-2.
Reduction in the odds of stroke and of coronary heart disease in the Hypertension Detection and Follow-up Program trial, the Medical Research Council trial, and in 12 other smaller, unconfounded randomized trials of antihypertensive therapy (mean diastolic blood pressure difference 5 to 6 mmHg for 5 years). (Collins R, Peto R, McMahon S, et al. *Lancet* 1990;335:833.)

vary randomly around zero. This assumption can be tested using standard statistical tests. An example of a well-known meta-analysis is shown in Figure 4-2. The question under study is whether lowering blood pressure with drugs will prevent the occurrence of strokes and coronary heart disease (CHD). In this meta-analysis, 14 studies with similar aims and event ascertainment are pooled. Observational studies would predict that a 5- to 6-mmHg difference in diastolic pressure between treatment and control should result in a 35% to 40% reduction in stroke and a 20% to 25% reduction in CHD. The meta-analysis shown in the figure illustrates that the observed reduction in strokes from this meta-analysis was 42%, actually more than predicted, but the reduction in CHD was only 14%, considerably less than predicted. This meta-analysis involves pooling 14 studies with nearly 37,000 patients. Any of the studies taken individually would be far too small and lack statistical power for observing this outcome. Meta-analysis is a powerful technique for analyzing data across studies. However, meta-analysis may sometimes overestimate value of treatment as a result of publication bias, which usually favors positive results because negative studies have less chance of being published and then included within the meta-analysis.

EPIDEMIOLOGIC REASONING

Establishing causation is an illusive but highly desirable goal in epidemiology and medicine. Once causation is established, changing the causative factor may be possible and the disease prevented. Causality is usually established by large-scale clinical trials. However, causation can also be inferred from epidemiologic observational data by applying several criteria (Table 4-1).

Strength

Observed relationships that are strong are more likely to be causal.

Graded (Dose) Response

Is the suspect factor related to graded (or dose) response to the disease? In other words, if one increases the exposure, does the disease risk increase? Factors not related to the disease in a graded fashion are probably not causative.

Independence

Does the suspect causal factor have a strong relationship to the disease and is it working directly to influence the disease, or is it merely associated with another factor that is the direct cause? For example, an early observation was that sugar consumption and CHD are strongly related. However, it is also true that high sugar consumers have heavier fat intakes. When one examines CHD in sugar consumers who have lower fat intake, no increased risk was observed. Therefore, one can conclude that sugar consumption is not independently associated with CHD; rather, it reflects a surrogate measure of fat consumption, which is *independently* associated with CHD.

TABLE 4-1.

Epidemiologic Factors for Inferring Causation from Observational Data

Strength
Graded (dose) response
Independence
Temporality
Specificity
Consistency/Congruence
Biologic plausibility

Temporality

Does the exposure *precede* the development of the disease? Only factors that precede the development of the disease are possible causes of the disease. For example, high blood cholesterol precedes the development of CHD; however, low blood cholesterol usually follows the development of cancer. In other words, high blood cholesterol causes CHD; cancer probably causes low blood cholesterol. In the former, cholesterol is the *cause* of the disease; in the latter, the *consequence* of the disease.

Specificity

Is the risk factor suspected of causing the disease specific for the disease or is it also associated with many other diseases? Again, high blood cholesterol is specific for risk of development of cardiovascular disease. Low blood cholesterol is associated not only with cancer death but also with death resulting from stroke, cirrhosis, lung disease, and AIDS, among others. Low blood cholesterol is nonspecific and less likely to be a cause of these diseases.

Consistency and Congruence

Has the factor under examination as a cause of the disease also been found to be related to the disease in other similar studies? Factors that are consistently related to the disease across a number of studies involving different populations are more likely to be causative. Furthermore, factors that are found to be related to the disease in some studies but not others are suspect. Again, high blood cholesterol as a risk factor for heart disease has been consistently shown in many studies carried out all over the world, whereas low blood cholesterol as a cause of cancer risk has not been found in several studies.

Are there other fields of investigation that support the relationship? For example, are there animal studies that manipulate the factor and find an association with the disease? Are there clinical studies consistent with the finding? Those factors that are congruent or "hold together" with other fields of investigation are more likely to be causative.

Biologic Plausibility

Is there a biologic mechanism known or hypothesized whereby the risk factor may cause the disease? Biologic plausibility is a powerful force in inferring causation. For example, it was observed for years that a minor fraction of blood lipids and lipoproteins—the high-density lipoprotein (HDL) cholesterol—was *inversely* related to CHD risk. This observation was counterintuitive: increased cholesterol caused cardiovascular disease, not decreased the risk. This fact was essentially ignored until a biologic mechanism was proposed whereby HDL cholesterol could act as the clearance mechanism of the body for excess cholesterol. Once this mechanism was proposed, decreased HDL cholesterol was further investigated and later accepted as a major causative factor for cardiovascular diseases.

These several criteria are useful not only in epidemiology but also in interpreting clinical studies and in clinical medicine. They provide a systematic construct to infer the likelihood of causation.

EVALUATING DIAGNOSTIC TESTS

The physician is faced with an almost continuous introduction of new diagnostic tests. New tests are frequently highly technical and expensive. It is important that new tests be evaluated against established tests to determine their practical value and cost-benefit.

A frequent approach to this evaluation is to establish the sensitivity and specificity of the new test against the established or "gold standard" test. The gold standard is the best test currently used to establish the presence of the disease.

Two kinds of errors are commonly made when a new test is conducted. If a test is negative when done on a patient known to have the disease, it is called a **false-negative.** If a test is positive and the patient does not have the disease, this is referred to as a **false-positive.** A test that is positive on patients with the disease is a **true-positive,** and a negative test in a person free of the disease is a **true-negative.** These values are used to determine the sensitivity and specificity of a test. **Sensitivity** is defined as the proportion of positive tests in patients who have the disease, or:

$$\frac{\text{True Positives}}{\text{True Positives} + \text{False Negatives}}$$

Specificity is defined as the proportion of correct assessments in persons without the disease, or:

$$\frac{\text{True Negatives}}{\text{True Negatives} + \text{False Positives}}$$

The positive **predictive value** of a test is the percentage of true positives of all the positives:

$$\frac{\text{True Positives}}{\text{True Positives} + \text{False Positives}}$$

A theoretic example is provided in Figure 4-3, which shows congestive heart failure (CHF) and the test (chest x-ray) cardiomegaly with a cardiothoracic ratio of greater than or equal to 0.5 on standard chest radiograph. Note in the example that the predictive value of the test has moderate positives associated with it.

	Patients Without CHF	Patients With CHF
Negative Test (Normal x-ray)	True Negative (TN) 1033	False Negative (FN) 50
Positive Test (Increased Cardiothoracic Ratio)	False Positive (FP) 104	True Positive (TP) 273

$$\text{Sensitivity} = \frac{TP}{TP + FN} = \frac{273}{273+50} = .85$$

$$\text{Specificity} = \frac{TN}{TN + FP} = \frac{1033}{1033 +104} = .91$$

$$\text{Predictive Value} = \frac{TP}{TP + FP} = \frac{273}{273+104} = 72\%$$

Figure 4-3.
Diagnostic sensitivity and specificity for diagnosing congestive heart failure by chest radiograph.

Some diagnostic tests can detect the presence of disease long before the patient becomes clinically ill (e.g., positive human immunodeficiency virus [HIV] test). Frequently, it is beneficial to detect disease early, especially if treatments are available that will cure the disease (e.g., mammography detects breast cancer, which is treatable under most circumstances if detected early). Such tests are frequently used to screen the population to detect early disease. It is very important with screening tests to establish the sensitivity, specificity, and predictive value of the test.

COMMUNICABLE DISEASES

The early development of epidemiology evolved primarily out of the study of infectious diseases. Although huge progress has been made in modern ability to diagnose and treat infections, formidable challenges remain. Infectious agents include bacteria, viruses, fungi, and parasites. In 1900, there were no effective treatments for infectious agents, and deaths occurring at birth and childhood were extremely common. In a family with 10 children, it was not unusual for five or more to die during childhood. Control efforts at that time were mainly isolation and quarantine. When it later became apparent that many new cases result from contact with asymptomatic carriers, these control methods were largely abandoned. High childhood mortality rates continue to be a serious problem within developing nations where infectious diseases remain a formidable public health problem.

Infections continue to plague developing countries. Each infectious disease is reported for individual illnesses or organisms, but because of underreporting, the total reported cases of infectious disease are invariably fewer than the true incidence. Infectious diseases are a common cause of visits to physicians' offices and for absences from work and school. Moreover, **nosocomial infections,** which are acquired in patient care facilities, affect millions of persons each year in the United States.

The spread of an infection increases directly with the number of existing cases, the number of susceptible persons, and a **transmission parameter.** The latter involves ease of transmission and relates to season, probability of contracting the infection, duration of infectivity, and frequency of subclinical infection. If a single case introduced into a real population causes no new infections, then no epidemic will occur. In most developed countries, for example, cases of measles stop reproducing when 94% of the population has become immune. Producing this level of immunity is regarded as feasible in the United States and Canada, where national elimination of measles is the officially adopted objective for measles control efforts.

Factors that are crucial to controlling the spread of infectious diseases from a public health point of view include (1) using methods to improve host resistance, such as using vaccinations, good nutrition, and good hygiene, (2) making efforts to reduce risk by altering the environment, such as cleaning the drinking water and testing blood products before use, and (3) using improved medical treatments via the health care system.

The problem of communicable disease results from a complex interplay between the host and the environment. The pathogenic microbe is necessary but not sufficient for clinical disease to occur. The extent of the problem is a complex interaction between a multitude of risk factors and the host.

New control measures have resulted from increased knowledge of the sources and modes of transmission of disease and from improved treatment methods. However, the evolution of new pathogens and the development of resistance continue to be problems.

An excellent source of up-to-date information on communicable diseases is the CDC's *Mortality and Morbidity Weekly Report* (MMWR).

EMERGING INFECTIONS

In recent years, there has been an emergence of bacteria and viruses that are resistant to antibiotic and antiviral therapy. These "superbugs" are a major public health concern. Resistant bacteria that have been isolated include staphylococcal, streptococcal, and pneumococcal pathogens. The indiscriminate use and overuse of antibiotics by physicians in the past have played a big role in the emergence of resistance. A major challenge for the infectious disease and pharmaceutical community is to develop new treatments in a timely manner so that new drugs will be available for treating these evolving pathogens. Furthermore, the indiscriminate "shotgun" use of antibiotics needs to be stopped.

Although tremendous progress has been made in their treatment and prevention, infectious diseases remain a major health concern and cause of death. Opportunities for infections to occur have increased with modern technologic advances. Immunosuppression in transplant patients, diseases that impair patients immunologically, implantation of artificial limbs, implantation of pacemakers, and increased exposure from worldwide travel are some of the current factors that have helped maintain infectious diseases as an important health concern. Immunosuppression increases risk for unusual opportunistic infections such as *Pneumocystis carinii* pneumonia, Kaposi's sarcoma, and cryptosporidiosis.

Epidemiologic methods and improved laboratory techniques have helped identify previously unknown entities, such as infection with HIV, the spirochete *Borrella burgdorferi* (Lyme disease), and hepatitis C. In addition, many diseases that were previously under control that were rare are again becoming a problem as a result of the emergence of resistant organisms. Examples include tuberculosis, rheumatic fever, staphylococcal infection, and cholera. Much of this emergence in resistance is due to the past overuse of antibiotics.

For infection to occur, the host must come into contact with the infectious organism. Several factors are involved in determining the likelihood of disease and its severity. Some of these factors include age, sanitation and personal hygiene, nutritional status, comorbidities, environment (work, home, leisure), geographic location, immunologic status, and climate.

Infections acquired at patient care facilities are called nosocomial infections. The risk of acquiring a nosocomial infection is greater at both inpatient and outpatient medical care facilities than it is elsewhere because medical care sites have more pathogens, use more invasive procedures, use immunosuppressive agents, and have a higher prevalence of drug-resistant pathogens.

In developed countries, control of infectious diseases is the dominant reason life expectancy increased dramatically in the 20th century; however, in developing countries, infectious diseases are still a burden that account for shorter life expectancy.

Much of the progress made combating infectious diseases can be attributed to widespread use of immunizations. Table 4-2 lists common infectious diseases and shows the dramatic reduction from the peak year of the infectious agent compared to 1992.

Vaccination is the delivery or administration of vaccine, a suspension of live attenuated or killed microorganism given to induce immunity and prevent infections. Immunization is the process of transferring immunity to the host. Immunization can be active or passive. An example of **active immunization** is injection of attenuated virus into the host, producing an endogenous immune response by the host. **Passive immunization** provides temporary protection through injection of prepared exogenous substances, such as immunoglobulin.

An important public health principle of immunization is herd immunity. Herd immunization occurs when the disease is effectively prevented in the population without 100% of individuals being vaccinated against the infection. Infectious organisms generally require a

TABLE 4-2.				
Comparison of Maximum and Current Morbidity for Vaccine-Preventable Diseases				

	Maximum Cases	Year	1992	Percentage Change
Diphtheria	206,939	1921	4	−99.99
Measles	894,134	1941	2237	−99.75
Mumps[a]	152,209	1968	2572	−98.31
Pertussis	265,269	1934	4083	−98.46
Polio (paralytic)	21,269	1952	4[b]	−99.98
Rubella[c]	57,686	1969	160	−99.72
CRS[d]	20,000	1964–1965	11	−99.95
Tetanus[e]	1,560	1923	45	−97.12
Haemophilus influenzae type b	20,000[f]	1984	1412	−92.94
Hepatitis B	26,611	1985	16,126	−39.40

[a]*First reportable in 1968.*

[b]*Subject to change as a result of retrospective case evaluation or late reporting.*

[c]*First reportable in 1966.*

[d]*Congenital rubella syndrome estimated for the 1964–1965 pandemic.*

[e]*Cases first reportable in 1947. Maximum based on number of deaths.*

[f]*First reportable in 1991. Estimate based on five US population-based studies, 1976–1984.*

certain level of person-to-person contact of nonimmunized people for transmission to occur. Once a certain prevalence of immunity is present, it is very difficult for the organism to be transmitted. Herd immunization allows for effective prevention of diseases in the population without having to achieve 100% immunization. Because of herd immunization and aggressive vaccination campaigns conducted in developed nations by government, schools, and health care organizations, many infectious diseases such as poliomyelitis, diphtheria, and tetanus only occur rarely, and **smallpox has been totally eradicated.** In developing nations where there is lack of financial resources and community organization, these same diseases are common.

To maintain herd immunization it is necessary to vaccinate each new generation. More and more school systems are mandating that vaccinations be a condition for attending school. Table 4-3 provides a recommended vaccination schedule for children from the Centers for Disease Control.

Influenza can infect elderly persons as well as younger persons with chronic cardiopulmonary disability, often resulting in hospitalization and complications. Antibody to the virus antigens reduces attack rates and the severity of infection. Because of the frequent change in the antigens, however, the most recent vaccine must be used, usually available each year in autumn. In 1987, only about 20% of the high-risk population in the United States had been immunized, creating continued annual health problems for the American population.

During an epidemic of influenza type A, amantadine helps kill the virus in individuals who have not received influenza vaccine. Amantadine is highly effective in preventing influenza type A in non-immunized persons, but side effects such as insomnia, dizziness, and personality changes may occur.

TABLE 4-3.

Recommended Schedule for Active Immunization of Normal Infants and Children

Recommended Age[a]	Vaccine(s)[b]	Comments
Birth	HBV[c]-1	Can be administered on discharge from the hospital
1–2 months	HBV-1 or HBV-2	Give HBV-1 if not administered at birth
2 months	DTP-1[d], OPV-1[e], Hib-1[f]	DTP can be given earlier (6 weeks) in areas of high endemicity for pertussis
4 months	DTP-2, OPV-2, Hib-2, HBV-2	6-week to 2-month interval desired between OPV doses to prevent interference. HBV-2 should be administered if not given earlier
6 months	DTP-3, Hib-3[g], OPV-3	OPV-3 customarily given at 15–18 months in the past
6–18 months	HBV-3	
12–15 months	MMR[h], Hib-3 or Hib-4	
15–18 months	DTP-4[i]	DTaP can be used in place of DTP
4–6 years	DTP-5[i], OPV-4, MMR-2[k]	At or before school entry. DTaP can be used in place of DTP
14–16 years	Td[l]	Repeat every 10 years throughout life

[a]These recommended ages should not be construed as absolute (i.e., 2 months can be 6–10 weeks). However, MMR should generally not be given to children younger than 1 year of age. Single measles antigen vaccine can be administered as early as 6 months of age if exposure to measles disease is considered likely. MMR can be used for infants if measles vaccine is unavailable.

[b]For all products used, consult the manufacturer's package enclosure for instructions regarding storage, handling, dosage, and administration. Immunobiologics prepared by different manufacturers can vary, and those of the same manufacturer can change from time to time. The package insert is a useful reference for a specific product, but it may not always be consistent with ACIP and AAP immunization schedules.

[c]Hepatitis B vaccine: can be given at birth, 1–2 months, and 6–18 months or 1–2 months, 4 months, and 6–18 months.

[d]DTP: diphtheria and tetanus toxoids and whole-cell pertussis vaccine adsorbed. DTP may be used up to the 7th birthday. The first dose can be given at 6 weeks of age and the second and third doses at 4–8 weeks after the preceding dose.

[e]OPV: Poliovirus vaccine live oral, trivalent; contains poliovirus types 1, 2, and 3. Doses of OPV should be separated by 6–8 week intervals.

[f]Haemophilus b conjugate vaccines.

[g]Hib-3 only needed if using the HbOC or PRP-T preparations. Unnecessary if using PRP-OMP.

[h]MMR: measles, mumps, and rubella virus vaccine, live. Hib-3 is indicated when using PRP-OMP, Hib-4 is indicated when using PRP-T of HbOC. MMR, Hib, and DTP can all be given together at 15 months.

[i]Provided at least 6 months has elapsed since DTP-3 or, if fewer than three DTPs have been received, at least 6 weeks since last previous dose of DTP. MMR vaccine should not be delayed to allow simultaneous administration with DTP and OPV. DTaP is diphtheria and tetanus toxoids and acellular pertussis vaccine.

[j]Up to the 7th birthday.

[k]The second dose of MMR can also be administered at entry to middle or junior high school, approximately 12 years of age.

[l]Td: tetanus and diphtheria toxoids adsorbed (for adult use); contains the same dose of tetanus toxoid as DTP or DT and a reduced dose of diphtheria toxoid.

(From Centers for Disease Control and Prevention.)

SURVEILLANCE AND CONTROL OF INFECTIOUS DISEASES

Education and information tend to be more acceptable to the public and less controversial than governmental legislation and regulation. Thus, groups in the United States continue to debate how strongly to enforce existing school immunization programs that have created immunization levels for most areas of the United States to levels that are the envy of other developed countries. Lowered levels of immunization in the United Kingdom, despite its national health service, relate partly to the greater reluctance among the British to use legal measures to get them done. In recent years, the frequency of tetanus has shifted markedly into older age groups. Case fatality ratios for tetanus are greater than 50% in persons older than 60 years; about half of all persons at these ages lack the protective antibody against tetanus toxin. Because many patients have not received a primary series of either tetanus or diphtheria toxoid, all adults who have not received a primary series of either tetanus or diphtheria toxoids should complete a series with the combined vaccine. Booster doses are then given every 10 years.

As preventable infections have become less frequent, the rare adverse effects of immunization have been increasingly publicized. A major source of this adverse publicity was an increased risk of Guillain-Barré syndrome caused by the influenza vaccine given in 1976; the vaccines of subsequent years have not resulted in similar risks, but the public reaction has not subsided entirely. The risk of lawsuits for compensation of those injured by immunization has hampered these preventive services and considerably raised the price of the vaccines. Thus, a maintenance system is needed to deliver routine immunization services without financial barriers in all health care settings. Medicare and Medicaid services cover the cost of influenza and pneumonia vaccines to older patients as long as the health care providers and institutions do not charge for them.

SEXUALLY TRANSMITTED DISEASES

For years, the primary targets of prevention programs for sexually transmitted diseases (STDs) were gonorrhea and syphilis. The spectrum expanded in the 1970s to include trichomoniasis, genital herpes, hepatitis, genital warts, and others. In the 1980s, AIDS was added to the list (see Chapter 9).

Identification and surveillance of STDs have been particularly difficult because of high carrier rates in asymptomatic persons. Moreover, diagnostic tests are expensive, and the national reporting systems have been weak. Women and children bear an inordinate share of STD complications: pelvic inflammatory disease, sterility, ectopic pregnancy, infant pneumonia, fetal and infant deaths, and infant mental retardation. Like other infections, STDs disproportionately affect the poor. Stronger financial support and adequate specialized clinics and programs are required to control and prevent these diseases. STDs are a huge problem in developing nations of the world.

More sustained and effective health education programs must aim at high-risk groups. When legislation decreased classroom education regarding STDs, there was a trend toward increased incidence of venereal disease among teenagers; when the legislation was rescinded, the disease trends reversed. In the most common of all STDs in the United States, trichomoniasis caused by *Chlamydia trachomatis*, the high cost and difficulty of detection have resulted in recommending the treatment of presumptive cases despite the lack of confirmation of diagnosis; in 70% of such cases, patients are asymptomatic. Condoms, when properly used during sexual activity, are the best known measure to avoid acquiring or transmitting many of the STDs.

Chapter 5

Evidence-Based Medicine

The primary task of physicians is to diagnose and treat disease. Historically (at least for the past 50 years), medical treatments have been primarily based on the state of knowledge concerning physiology and biochemistry and related mechanistic pathways. These mechanistic-derived clinical paradigms have usually been based on research involving animal models approximating human disease. Analogous disease surrogates were developed in animals to best fit human diseases (e.g., salt-sensitive hypertension in rat models based on the renin-angiotensin pathway).

The development of these models and mechanistic pathways has been very useful, especially for diagnostic pattern recognition and prognosis, by helping to describe the clinical natural history of the disease. However, for developing effective treatments for various diseases in humans, the mechanistic paradigm has had limitations.

One problem is that most mechanistic pathways are much more complicated than theorized, involving numerous interrelated pathways, many of which are unknown. Also, animal disease models differ from human diseases and only rarely can the results be directly extrapolated. Finally, the disease-oriented mechanistic paradigm primarily focuses on patients with the disease, and knowledge is limited regarding those people who do not get the disease or who do not receive treatment (or for whom treatment is not available). Out of necessity, physicians historically have selected treatments mainly by using "clinical judgment," intuitive reasoning based on their own and on their superiors' experiences in treating disease.

Evidence-based medicine is an emerging discipline that advocates that, whenever possible, treatment regimens be based on scientifically sound evidence carried out on human participants. The primary tool for evidence-based medicine is the **clinical trial.** Clinical trials compare treatments with controls that consist of no treatment, placebo, or other treatment (standard care).

Because the science of clinical trials is relatively new and the method is comparatively expensive, clinical trial data for most diseases are either nonexistent or represented by a number of small studies that usually vary considerably in design and quality. To partially address this limitation, an analysis method for trial results has been developed called **meta-analysis.** In this analysis, the study itself is the analytic unit. Figure 4-2 (see Chapter 4) shows a well-known meta-analysis that addresses the following question: Does lowering diastolic pressure by 5 to 6 mmHg with drugs prevent stroke and coronary heart disease (CHD)? The results show that, overall, in the treated group with lower pressures, the occurrence of stroke was reduced by 42% and CHD by 14%, both statistically significant results. This was the first time that it was shown convincingly that reducing blood pressure prevents CHD. Prior studies were insufficiently powered (too small) to provide a clear answer to this question. Subsequent trial results have verified this meta-analysis.

Meta-analyses are very useful, but this method also has limitations. Decisions must be made on what criteria to use to select studies to be included. Positive studies are more likely to be published and easier to find, and locating all relevant studies is difficult. Furthermore, individual studies usually differ in terms of types of patients, measurements, and protocol.

Recently, several large clinical studies with large sample sizes have reported results that differ from previous meta-analyses. This is mostly a reflection of the problems with meta-analysis. The results of one or two sufficiently powered (large enough), well-conducted clinical trials are preferable to meta-analyses for making recommendations for treatments.

The discipline of evidence-based medicine is rapidly developing. More and more, trials are being conducted and the outcomes held up as the "gold standard" for evaluating treatments. This increased interest can be attributed in part to the increasing costs of health care. Physicians can no longer afford the luxury of prescribing widespread treatments that have not been scientifically evaluated. For this reason, the field of evidence-based medicine will continue to grow.

Chapter 6

Managed Care

Managed care refers to organizational relationships between health plans and physicians which provide medical care at a lower cost. Organizational elements of managed care are designed to reduce use of health care practices, which, in turn, holds down costs.

Managed care programs, particularly health maintenance organizations (HMOs), began in the late 1950s and have greatly proliferated. By 1995, the majority of adults in the United States with health insurance used some form of managed care. The concept of managed care arose and proliferated in response to rapidly increasing health care costs, which were escalating at a much higher rate than overall inflation. Common forms of managed care include HMO staff models, with physicians employed as salaried employees of the plan; preferred provider organizations, in which physicians contract with one or more plans to deliver care in their clinic; and capitation plans, in which a health plan contracts with a business or Medicare/Medicaid for a specific prepaid per patient fee to provide care. If the health plan provides care that is more costly than the amount negotiated, the financial loss is the responsibility of the health plan. Managed care plans can be either nonprofit or for-profit organizations.

MANAGING COSTS

Managed care has used three main methods to contain costs: gatekeeper systems, physician incentives, and utilization review.

Gatekeepers

The gatekeeper concept is designed to limit patient contacts with specialist physicians, because specialist visits tend to be much more costly than primary care visits. Patients must see their primary care "gatekeeper" first to determine whether referral to a specialist is appropriate. This method reduces substantially specialist referrals. Specialists tend to order more costly laboratory tests and to prescribe newer (and usually more expensive) medications. Gatekeepers are usually primary care physicians, most often family practitioners and internists. Gatekeepers approve or disapprove the referral to a specialist. Primary care gatekeepers make the decisions that determine health care utilization. Some managed care plans allow direct access to specialists, but patients pay a higher premium or copayment for this access.

Physician Incentives

Physician incentives, which could also be viewed as disincentives, usually take the form of withholding a portion of the annual salary and providing periodic "bonuses" for remaining within cost guidelines. For example, a physician may order fewer diagnostic tests, fewer patients may be hospitalized, and fewer patients may make clinic visits. Incentives have almost always rewarded less utilization. Capitation can be viewed as a form of incentive to see fewer patients. Ethics is a major consideration with incentives, with most plans considering that disclosure to the patient of the incentive relationship is essential, even though sometimes plans try to prevent such disclosure.

Utilization Review

Utilization review takes the form of precertification for surgical and other high-cost procedures, nurse chart abstracting, second opinions, and case management. This method essentially sets "rules" and treatment referral algorithms that are designed to restrict use of high cost and sometimes unnecessary procedures.

MANAGED CARE: STRENGTHS AND WEAKNESSES

Managed care has had many positive aspects, including a track record of reducing the rate of increase in health care costs and providing improved data systems for systematic analysis of health care delivery. In a few areas, managed care has succeeded in emphasizing prevention of disease. To date, managed care has successfully reduced utilization of higher cost and higher risk procedures.

As managed care has evolved, several problems have become apparent. Incorporation of managed care has shifted primary responsibility for the patient from the individual physician to "the plan." The plan is then responsible for thousands of "lives covered." The basic relationship between the physician and the patient has been significantly altered. Continuity of care has been deemphasized as patients and physicians move among carriers and plans. The average stay in a managed care plan is 2 to 3 years.

For-profit managed care and capitation have resulted in a short-range view that emphasizes decreased utilization and reduced staffing over a longer view that stresses prevention of disease. Because quality of care is difficult to define and expensive to measure, to date, emphasis has been placed primarily on the process of capitation and utilization review. Patients' trust levels in their physicians and medical plans have declined. In some instances, the doctor-patient communication is also impaired because some plans encourage their physicians not to communicate utilization rules to patients.

In 1998, forty million Americans had no health care insurance. Moving into the 21st century, the health care system and managed care face many challenges:

1. How can health care costs be controlled in an environment of rapidly evolving technology, which constantly produces new and usually more expensive drugs and devices?
2. Many responsibilities formerly provided by government or medical schools are viewed as money losers. Who will be responsible for funding and conducting medical education and training? In general, managed care has been reluctant to take on these tasks.
3. What are the legal implications for the plan that controls physician behavior using negative incentives and utilization review and that holds the physician responsible for malpractice claims?
4. How can quality care be emphasized?
5. How will plans adapt to legislation that increasingly limits health care legislation?

These are some of the important questions that must be addressed as the American health care system addresses rapid changes.

Chapter 7

Health Services Research

In 1995, the Institute of Medicine defined health services research as follows: "Health services research is a multidisciplinary field of inquiry, both basic and applied, that examines the use, costs, quality, accessibility, delivery, organization, financing, and outcomes of health care services to increase knowledge and understanding of the structure, processes and effects of health services for individuals and populations." In addition to the traditional biomedical fields, the multidisciplinary nature of health services research draws upon the skills of a diverse range of academic disciplines including epidemiology, biostatistics, sociology, and economics. If all health research were organized on a continuum, it might start at the molecular end with the basic sciences of biology, chemistry, and physics. Further along the continuum would be bench research, in which experiments are conducted and observations are made in test tubes and laboratory animals, and clinical biomedical research, which uses consenting human subjects. The continuum would embrace health services research, with some overlap at the point where clinical research begins to answer questions about what works best in real practice settings and in the community. Outcomes research and cost-effectiveness trials tend to focus on clinical interventions for individual patients, whereas guidelines and technology assessments address systems and populations. At the community end of the continuum, health services researchers study how medical care is organized and financed.

The scope of health services research can perhaps best be appreciated by citing several key themes with relevant examples of actual studies in each key area. These themes are summarized in Table 7-1.

Clinical evaluation and outcomes research look at the benefits and harms of alternative strategies for preventing, diagnosing, and treating illness. Whereas traditional clinical trials typically examine **"efficacy"** of interventions **(benefit under ideal conditions),** outcomes research most often examines **"effectiveness"** of interventions **(benefit under typical practice conditions).**

Some types of outcomes research resemble a traditional clinical trial except that **effectiveness rather than efficacy is the outcome of interest.** For example, the efficacy of nicotine replacement for smoking cessation was first demonstrated using highly trained staff who provided advice and support to highly motivated volunteers. The effectiveness of nicotine replacement was later demonstrated under

TABLE 7-1.

Key Themes of Health Services Research

Clinical evaluation and outcomes research
Informatics and clinical decision making
Practitioner, patient, and consumer behavior
Quality of care
Access to health care
Health profession's work force
Organization and financing of health services

typical office practice conditions with average smokers. Most often, however, for practical reasons, outcomes research is observational rather than experimental. For example, New York State has an ongoing system to monitor the mortality rate of patients undergoing coronary artery bypass grafting, and comparisons are made between different surgeons and hospitals or systems of care.

Informatics and clinical decision making is the study of how timely access to accurate information about treatment options and outcomes affects the decision-making process of both patients and physicians. Rapidly evolving technologies are stimulating much exciting new research. For example, clinical information systems and electronic medical records are being used to help physicians make wiser and more cost-effective antibiotic choices for treating infections. Interactive computer software has been developed to guide patients through complex decisions such as whether to undergo coronary artery bypass grafting or angioplasty for coronary artery atherosclerosis, PSA testing to screen for prostatic cancer, and transurethral resection of the prostate for prostatic hypertrophy.

Studies of practitioners, patients, and consumer behavior regarding health care are important areas of health services research. For example, for the practitioner, this includes studies of how specialty training, practice environment, or economic incentives affect the provision of health care services. Another example is the study of how copayments influence patients' decisions about seeking both discretionary and nondiscretionary health care.

Questions about how quality of care affects health care outcomes have been increasingly voiced by the public and policy makers during the recent upheavals in health care organization. Much work has been done to develop the basic tools to define and measure both quality of care and disease-specific functional outcomes. For example, the Health Employee Data and Information Set (HEDIS) is an attempt to standardize the measures of performance so that meaningful comparisons can be made between health plans. Earlier versions of HEDIS were limited to such easily quantifiable outcomes as the rate of mammography and completeness of childhood immunization. More recent versions of HEDIS have been expanded to include more numerous and complex measures, and to address both the process as well as the outcome of care.

Access to health care, or the timely receipt of appropriate health care, is another focus of health services research, which has been attracting increased public attention. Recent findings, for example, that African Americans have lower rates of coronary revascularization and kidney transplantation compared to white patients raise numerous questions about the root causes of these differences.

The composition of the health profession workforce is critical to efforts to plan for the future health care system in the United States. For example, health services researchers in this area ask questions about the optimal ratio of providers to patients, generalists to specialists, and physicians to "physician extenders" (e.g., nurse practitioners). Other important topics include geographic maldistribution of health care providers and the related issue of how international medical graduates fit into the U.S. health care system.

The organization and financing of health care services, one of the most contentious policy issues in the United States, falls within the purview of health services research. An excellent example is the Medical Outcome Study, an observational study of outcomes in hypertensive and diabetic patients cared for in three different systems of care (HMOs, large multispecialty groups, and solo or single-specialty groups) by generalist and subspecialist physicians. Although randomized trials in this area are unusual, the Hennepin County Medicaid Demonstration Project compared the processes and outcomes of care for a variety of conditions ranging from diabetes to mental illness in Medicaid recipients randomly allocated to capitated versus fee-for-service care.

Chapter 8

Ethnicity

Race is a commonly used descriptor in medicine and public health, as well as in society. This term is usually used to describe an individual patient in various medical settings, even when race or ethnicity does not contribute substantively to medical decision making. The meaning of race is rarely defined, although its continued pervasive use suggests, at the very least, an implicit understanding of the societal and scientific implications of race. Race represents a social categorization that is primarily based on phenotype, with heavy reliance on skin tone differences. A common perception has been that racial identity represents intrinsic biologic differences attributable to unique genetic factors that lend validity to the partitioning of the human species into subspecies. The logic for this paradigm is, however, severely flawed.

Race is deeply intertwined with socioeconomic conditions, including income, nutrition (including prenatal), exposure to violent crime, psychosocial stressors, physical activity, and other lifestyle variables. Disentangling the influence of these and other environmental and lifestyle exposures from that of race is a daunting, if not impossible, task. Numerous examples of racial differentials in disease incidence and disease-specific mortality rates have been recognized (Figure 8-1). It is very difficult to formulate an intuitively appealing unifying genetic hypothesis to explain the excess mortality burden of African Americans relative to whites across this broad range of unrelated diseases.

Few diseases have been the focus of intense speculation regarding the causes of the racial differences in disease incidence, prevalence, and severity as it has in hypertension. Several environmental exposures and lifestyle attributes such as obesity and physical inactivity, known risk factors for hypertension, are more prevalent among African Americans (particularly women) than among whites. Accordingly, hypertension is more prevalent in African Americans, particularly African-American women, than in whites. Despite the presence of these and other well-defined environmental factors and lifestyle attributes, genetic factors have frequently been deemed responsible for the excess hypertension in African Americans compared to whites. The age-adjusted African-American/white blood pressure differential has narrowed considerably over the past 3 decades. The relatively short timeframe of the blood pressure convergence is most logically explained by changing environmental

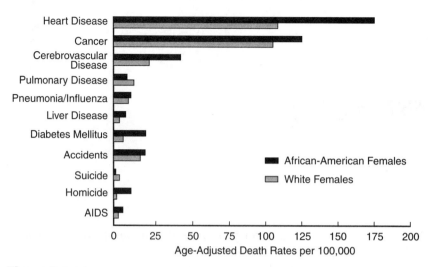

Figure 8-1.
African Americans have higher death rates than whites for most major causes of death. For almost all major causes of death, African Americans have higher age-adjusted death rates than whites. The data in this figure are for females in 1988, but the differences are even more pronounced for males. (Source: National Center for Health Statistics, 1991, Health, United States, 1990 [Hyattsville, MD: NCHS].)

rather than genetic factors. Hypertension is also associated inversely with socioeconomic standing in both African Americans and whites; therefore, it should not be surprising that some of the blood pressure differential present between African Americans and whites relates to the well-documented differences in income that have been shown to correlate with lifestyle and behavioral attributes that predispose to hypertension. Finally, race disease differentials are not static; thus, one racial group may have higher disease rates relative to another race at one point, but lower disease rates at another. Breast cancer is an example of such a flip-flop in disease rates between African Americans and whites.

Powerful molecular genetic tools have been developed that allow objective scientific inquiry, not only into the differences in disease burden between race and ethnic groups, but also to explain the variation of disease rates within these groups. Cystic fibrosis is the most common lethal autosomal recessive disorder in Americans and is typically thought of as a disease affecting white populations exclusively. Approximately 750 genetic mutations of the CFTR gene, affecting multiple cell lines, have been identified with the del F508 mutation accounting for approximately 70% of the CFTR gene mutations. This mutation is more common in whites than in African Americans; however, this disease also affects African Americans. The remaining 30% of CFTR gene mutations are just as common in African Americans as in whites. African Americans show striking geographic differences in vascular disease susceptibility. However, many African Americans go undiagnosed, in part as a consequence of the lack of appreciation that this genetic disease affects them. For example, stroke risk is 30% to 40% higher in African Americans residing in the 13 southeastern states compared to African Americans residing elsewhere in the

United States. It is likely that environmental factors explain this difference. Nevertheless, genetic variation merits investigation as a potential contributor to this intraracial geographic vascular disease differential.

What has been the outcome of medical research being so focused on racial contrasts? First, factors that explain disease occurrence within an ethnic group may be overlooked because of the implicit assumption of homogeneity of disease expression within an ethnic group. An example of this is the recently defined link between body size and salt sensitivity in African Americans, an observation that is true in both African Americans and whites. Second, genetic differences are invoked to explain interracial differences in disease rates, often in the absence of any tangible evidence, thus lending an aura of inevitability to disease occurrences that could otherwise be modified by prudent lifestyle and behavior changes. Furthermore, genetic explanations for race differentials in disease have been detrimental because of the selective use of such explanations in diseases with a significant social stigma. The acquired immunodeficiency syndrome and other sexually transmitted diseases are notable examples in which African Americans have been negatively associated with a high incidence of disease. Such explanations tend to ignore the fact that race is only one variable by which individuals or groups can be classified, and the influences of other factors that may be associated with race are usually more logical explanations of the observed disease differentials. Even when potential confounders of the race-disease relationship are adjusted for in multivariate statistical models, inaccuracies in the measurement/ classification of independent variables, often socioeconomic factors, lead to residual confounding and thus an overestimate of the strength of the race-disease relationship. Third, important intraethnic variations in disease occurrence tend to be overlooked when inordinate focus is placed on interracial comparisons.

When interrace differentials in disease are observed, the most likely explanation for excess in one racial group relative to another relates to environmental influences. Among American blacks there is a tremendously diverse genetic gene pool, which spans the continent of Africa, the Caribbean, and Central/South America and includes whites. Among whites, a wide genetic diversity also exists. Thus it is hardly surprising that race does not equal genetic homogeneity because the genetic heterogeneity within ill-defined racial groups exceeds that present between racial groups. Thus, genetic factors are unlikely to explain racial differences in disease occurrence at the population level. The notion of race as a means of providing a biologic framework for classifying humans is a concept that is likely flawed and should be reconsidered.

Chapter 9

High Priority Areas for Community Medicine

Prevention and treatment are not mutually exclusive activities, although a number of health services tend to approach them in that fashion. Part of the effort in controlling rising costs of health care involves raising the priority of preventive services. In contrast to the relatively simple preventive measures such as giving immunizations, much prevention in the future will be long term, continuous, and aimed at improving the individual's knowledge about disease and health-related behavior patterns. The following sections discuss areas of prevention that will become areas of high priority in the coming years and that have important public health significance.

HIGH BLOOD PRESSURE

High blood pressure is the most prevalent medical condition in the United States. Approximately one in four adults has hypertension; it is the most common single reason for a patient to visit a primary care physician. Periodically, official groups develop guidelines for managing high blood pressure. Every 4 to 5 years in the United States, the Joint National Committee on the Prevention, Detection, Evaluation and Treatment of High Blood Pressure (JNC) publishes updated guidelines for defining and managing high blood pressure. The JNC is made up of national experts in the hypertensive field who are selected through the National High Blood Pressure Education Program of the National Heart Lung and Blood Institute (NHLBI). The sixth report (JNC VI) was published in 1997 in the *Archives of Internal Medicine* (volume 157, page 2413). These reports have been very influential, and the recommendations are used by many countries around the world.

Since the JNC reports were initiated, there has been a continuous trend to revise downward the levels of blood pressure that are of concern. Figure 9-1 and Table 9-1 provide data from the National Health and Nutrition Examination Surveys (NHANES) on aware-

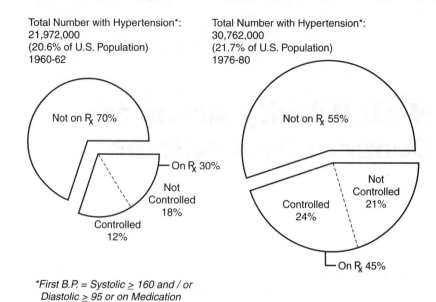

Total Number with Hypertension*:
21,972,000
(20.6% of U.S. Population)
1960-62

Total Number with Hypertension*:
30,762,000
(21.7% of U.S. Population)
1976-80

*First B.P. = Systolic ≥ 160 and / or
Diastolic ≥ 95 or on Medication

Figure 9-1.
The total number of hypertensive people in the United States aged 18 to 74 years, estimated from the National Health and Nutrition Examination Surveys of 1960 to 1962 and 1976 to 1980 and the percentages of those not on therapy, on therapy not controlled, and on therapy controlled. (*Arch Intern Med* 1993;153:160.)

ness, treatment, and control of high blood pressure in adults from the mid-1970s to the mid-1980s. In the mid-1980s, approximately one third of people with high blood pressure were unaware of their condition, only half underwent treatment, and only 24% had the disease under control (blood pressure [BP] <140 mmHg systolic or <90 mmHg diastolic). Data comparing phases 1 and 2 of NHANES III indicate that the level of blood pressure control in recent years is getting worse and not better. This is alarming because high blood pressure is relatively easy to diagnose and there are numerous effective treatments available to lower blood pressure and substantially prevent cardiovascular mortality and morbidity figures. Figure 9-2 shows the age-adjusted reduction in mortality rates from stroke

TABLE 9-1.

Findings of Three Hypertension Surveys Using Data from Persons 25 to 74 Years of Age

	National Health Survey (1960–1962)	National Health and Nutrition Examination Survey I (1971–1975)	National Health and Nutrition Examination Survey II (1976–1980)
No. of people examined	6,672	17,796	16,204
% with BP ≥160/95	20.3	22.1	22.0
% of hypertensives aware of diagnosis	49	64	73
% of hypertensives being treated	31	34	56
% of hypertensives under control	16	20	34

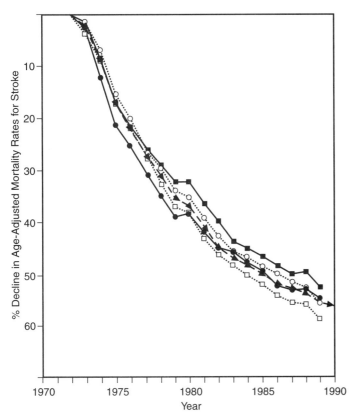

Figure 9-2.
Decline in age-adjusted mortality rate for stroke by race and gender since 1972. Triangles indicate total; solid squares, African-American men; solid circles, African-American women; open squares, white men; and open circles, white women. Data for 1990 are provisional. Race and gender data for 1990 were not yet available. (Source: National Center for Health Statistics data calculated by the National Heart, Lung and Blood Institute.)

since 1970 by ethnic gender subgroups. Although there has been an impressive decline, there is evidence that since the mid-1990s this decline has leveled out.

Systolic blood pressure is much more important than was previously thought. Fifteen-year follow-up data from more than 362,000 middle-aged men screened for eligibility into the Multiple Risk Factor Intervention Trial have shown that systolic blood pressure is a much more potent risk factor compared to diastolic blood pressure. Systolic blood pressure increases progressively with age (Figure 9-3), so systolic hypertension is a major problem in older people. Several studies have recently shown that lowering systolic blood pressure with drugs reduces rates of total stroke, coronary heart disease (CHD), and heart failure significantly (Figure 9-4).

Table 9-2 provides JNC V guidelines for adult (age 18 years of age and older) classification of blood pressure. Optimal blood pressure is less than 120 mmHg systolic and less than 80 mmHg diastolic. Hypertension is divided into four stages:

1. High normal: systolic blood pressure (SBP) 130 to 139/diastolic blood pressure (DBP) 85 to 89

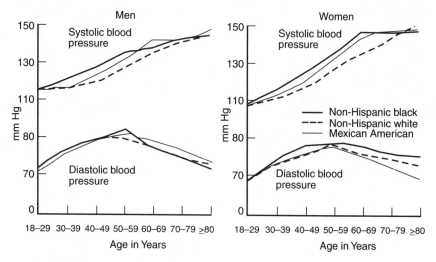

Figure 9-3.
Mean systolic and diastolic blood pressure by age and race/ethnicity for men and women aged 18 years and older in the United States.

2. Stage 1: SBP 140 to 159/DBP 90 to 99 mmHg
3. Stage 2: SBP 160 to 179/DBP 100 to 109 mmHg
4. Stage 3: SBP 180 or greater and/or DBP 110 mmHg or greater

A few recommendations from JNC VI base treatment recommendations not only on level of blood pressure but also on extent of cardiovascular risk. This approach is outlined in Tables 9–3 and 9–4. Hypertension is treated based on level of risk. Risk group A is low risk. Persons in this risk group only have high blood pressure and do not have other cardiovascular risk factors, target organ damage, or clinical cardiovascular disease (CVD). Risk group B is intermediate. Persons in

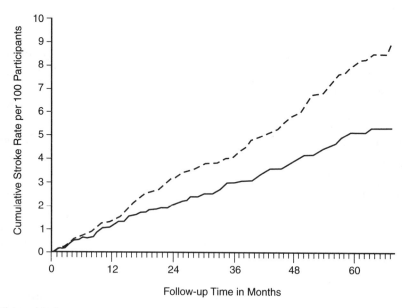

Figure 9-4.
Cumulative fatal plus nonfatal stroke rate per 100 participants in the active treatment (*solid line*) and placebo (*broken line*) groups during the Systolic Hypertension in the Elderly Program. (*JAMA* 1991;265:3255–3264. Copyright 1991, American Medical Association.)

TABLE 9-2.

Classification of Blood Pressure for Adults Age 18 Years and Older[a]

Category	Systolic (mmHg)	Diastolic (mmHg)
Normal[b]	<130	<85
High Normal[b]	130–139	85–89
Hypertension[c]		
Stage 1 (mild)	140–159	90–99
Stage 2 (moderate)	160–179	100–109
Stage 3 (severe)	180–209	110–119
Stage 4 (very severe)	≥210	≥120

[a]Not taking antihypertensive drugs and not acutely ill. When systolic and diastolic pressures fall into different categories, the higher category should be selected to classify the individual's blood pressure status. For instance, 160/92 mmHg should be classified as stage 2, and 180/120 mmHg should be classified as stage 4. Isolated systolic hypertension (ISH) is defined as SBP≥140 mmHg and DBP <90 mmHg and staged appropriately (e.g., 170/85 mmHg is defined as stage 2 ISH).

[b]Optimal blood pressure with respect to cardiovascular risk is SBP < 120 mmHg and DBP < 80 mmHg. However, unusually low readings should be evaluated for clinical significance.

[c]Based on the average of two or more readings obtained at each of two or more visits following an initial screening.

Note: In addition to classifying stages of hypertension based on average blood pressure levels, the clinician should specify presence or absence of target-organ disease and additional risk factors. For example, a patient with diabetes and a blood pressure of 142/94 mmHg plus left ventricular hypertrophy should be classified as "stage 1 hypertension with target-organ disease (left ventricular hypertrophy) and with another major risk factor (diabetes.)" This specificity is important for risk classification and management.

From the Fifth Report of the Joint National Committee on Detection, Evaluation, and Treatment of High Blood Pressure. NIH publication #93-1088, 1993.

this group do not yet have evidence of target organ damage or clinical CVD but do have one or more additional risk factors. Risk group C is the higher risk group and persons in this group require treatment based on the presence of target organ damage, clinical cardiovascular disease, or diabetes mellitus. Table 9-5 lists the major risk factors and target organ damage criteria required for this classification.

Lifestyle modification is recommended for prevention and treatment of high blood pressure. Lifestyle treatments include weight loss, reduction of dietary sodium and alcohol intake, and increased physical activity. Other potential lifestyle factors include increasing potassium, calcium, and magnesium intake, although these recommendations are not as strongly supported in well-designed studies.

The JNC VI recommends the following groups of agents as initial drug therapy: diuretics, beta blockers, calcium channel blockers, angiotensin-converting enzyme inhibitors, alpha blockers, and alpha-beta blockers. Diuretics and beta blockers are listed as preferred agents for the uncomplicated low risk group A because these

TABLE 9-3.

Cardiovascular Risk Grouping in Patients with Hypertension (JNC VI)

Risk Group	Blood Pressure	Risk Factors	Target Organ Damage/ Clinical Cardiovascular Disease
A	High	No other	Neither
B	High	At least one	Neither
C	High	At least one	One or both and/or diabetes mellitus

agents have been shown in clinical trials to lower CVD mortality and morbidity rates. Based on recent trial results from the Systolic Hypertension in Europe Study, long-acting dihydropyridine calcium blockers are also considered with diuretics and beta blockers as preferred in isolated systolic hypertension in elderly patients.

Three points emphasized by JNC VI are that (1) drugs with long half-lives or duration of action should be considered to lower blood pressure within 24 hours, (2) blood pressure drugs should be started at low doses and gradually titrated upward, and (3) combination drugs (two or more different types of blood pressure drugs in one pill) are acceptable in managing hypertension.

One of the main public health priorities is to improve diagnosis, treatment, and control of high blood pressure. More emphasis is also being placed on preventing high blood pressure through healthier living.

TABLE 9-4.

Cardiovascular Risk Stratification and Treatment in Patients with Hypertension (JNC VI)

Blood Pressure Stage (mmHg)	Risk Groups		
	A	B	C
High normal (130–139/85–89)	Lifestyle	Lifestyle	Drug treatment
Stage I (140–159/90–99)	Lifestyle	Lifestyle	Drug treatment
Stages II and III (≥130/≥100)	Drug treatment	Drug treatment	Drug treatment

> **TABLE 9-5.**
>
> **Components of Cardiovascular Risk Grouping in Patients with Hypertension (JNC VI)**
>
> **Major risk factors**
> Smoking
> Dyslipidemia
> Diabetes mellitus
> Age > 60 years
> Sex (men and postmenopausal women)
> Family history of cardiovascular disease (CVD)
>   Women < 65 years
>   Men <55 years
> **Target Organ Damage / Clinical CVD**
> Heart diseases
>   Left ventricular hypertrophy
>   Angina pectoris
>   Prior myocardial infarction
>   Prior coronary revascularization
>   Heart failure
> Stroke or transient ischemic attack
> Nephropathy
> Peripheral arterial disease
> Retinopathy

ACQUIRED IMMUNODEFICIENCY SYNDROME

Rare cases of acquired immunodeficiency syndrome (AIDS) have been documented using autopsy material from as far back as 1959. The first cases of AIDS as an identifiable syndrome were diagnosed in the United States in 1981. Over that decade, AIDS spread rapidly until it became a worldwide pandemic. Areas of the world that have been especially hard hit are sub-Saharan Africa, the Indian subcontinent, and Southeast Asia. Most cases of infection with human immunodeficiency virus (HIV) are caused by type I virus. Type II virus infections occur in Western Africa and are purported to be less severe. Initially, cases were primarily found in male homosexuals, intravenous drug users, blood transfusion patients, and hemophiliacs, and the transmission pattern suggested an infectious etiology. In 1983–1984, HIV was isolated and established as the agent of transmission. Screening tests for HIV antibodies were developed to assist the identification of asymptomatic carriers. HIV is a retrovirus that has a long incubation period of up to several years. The virus severely impairs the immune system and creates susceptibility to a variety of infections. Major concomitant diseases are *Pneumocystis carinii* pneumonia and Kaposi's sarcoma. In 1990, it was estimated that 1 to 2 million Americans were infected with HIV, and AIDS cases have steadily increased each year (Figure 9-5). The virus has been isolated from all body fluids, including blood, semen, saliva,

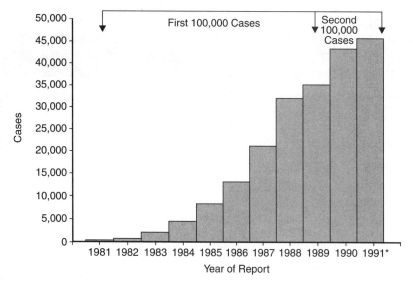

* Cases reported through December 1991.

Figure 9-5.
AIDS cases, by year of report—United States, 1981 to 1991. (*MMWR* 1992;41:28.)

tears, urine, breast milk, and cerebrospinal fluid. Major routes of transmission are through (1) sexual contact, especially anal intercourse among homosexual males and vaginal intercourse among heterosexuals, (2) intravenous drug use, (3) contaminated blood products, (4) perinatal contact of a fetus with an infected mother, and (5) breast milk, although this mode of infection is rare. There is no credible evidence that HIV is spread by casual contact. Even though heterosexual transmission in the United States accounts for only a small percentage of the total incidence, such transmission has been increasing at the fastest rate. In 1998 in the United States, the high-risk groups remain the same, with the most common being male homosexuals and intravenous drug users. **Infection from blood and blood product transfusions has become uncommon.** The incidence of transmission through heterosexual intercourse, however, is increasing. African Americans and Hispanics are at higher risk than are whites. Worldwide, heterosexual contact is the dominant means of infection, accounting for the equal ratio of infection among men and women in Africa and Asia.

AIDS patients are frequent users of health care, and hospital admissions are usually for treatment of opportunistic infectious diseases. In many large US cities, AIDS is the number one cause of death among men 25 to 44 years of age.

The most common modes of transmission for AIDS are through semen and blood, and a widespread AIDS education program aimed at promoting "safe sex" is in place. This program aims at persuading people to avoid high-risk sexual behavior, such as engaging in anal sex and promiscuity, and encourages the use of condoms. In the past, treatment for HIV infection has been limited. Azidothymidine, or AZT, was the first drug shown to be effective in palliative treatment and in prolonging remission in AIDS patients. In the United States, rapid gains have been made in the drug treatment of AIDS.

By the late 1990s, substantial progress was made in combating this HIV epidemic. Medical care has been improved, especially with antiretroviral therapy. Three drug regimens—protease inhibitors, nonnucleoside reverse transcriptase inhibitors, and nucleoside analogues—substantially slow the rate of disease progression. In 1996, the number of AIDS deaths declined (23%) for the first time in the United States; in 1998, the number of deaths decreased by 19% compared to 1997. This has been attributed largely to multidrug antiretroviral therapy. Most AIDS deaths are caused by opportunistic infections, that is, infections that occur as a result of the severe suppression of the immune system. HIV has an affinity for T lymphocytes, which it kills, bringing about a reduction in T helper lymphocytes (CD4 count). Lower levels of CD4 lymphocytes are an important surrogate predictor of opportunistic infections and death. *Pneumocystis carinii* pneumonia is the most common opportunistic infection occurring in AIDS patients. Figure 9-6 shows the incidence of HIV-opportunistic infection and deaths, showing the 1996 decline. Other important factors associated with HIV outcomes include overall health and nutritional status, repeated exposure to the virus, and route of infection.

Because of the prevention and treatment successes in the United States, it appears that the AIDS epidemic is coming under control, but it is important not to become complacent; HIV is able to mutate and become drug resistant. Worldwide, there is an HIV pandemic. In 1998, the World Health Organization estimated that there were 16,000 new cases of HIV infection every day. Certain areas of the world have an extremely high prevalence of HIV infection in the general population;

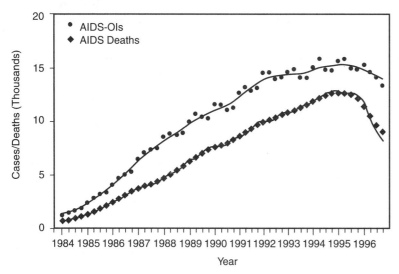

Figure 9-6.
Estimated incidence of AIDS-opportunistic illnesses (AIDS-OIs) and estimated number of deaths among persons aged 13 years of age and older with AIDS (AIDS deaths), adjusted for delays in reporting, by quarter year of diagnosis/death—United States, 1984 to 1996. Points represent quarterly incidence; lines represent "smoothed" incidence. Estimates are not adjusted for incomplete reporting of AIDS cases.

these areas are Central and East Africa, Southeast Asia, especially Thailand, and the Indian subcontinent. In these areas of the world, the AIDS pandemic is even more tragic because these countries have severe limitations on resources for the diagnosis, treatment, and prevention of HIV infection. In most of these areas, infected persons do not have access even to conventional medical care. To improve this crisis, a worldwide coordinated effort is needed. This approach includes (1) a national standard for reporting HIV infections, (2) better access to new HIV drugs, (3) referral of AIDS patients to physicians who are experienced in treating HIV infection, and (4) safeguards on maintaining privacy and minimizing discrimination. It is hoped that a vaccine can be developed to minimize HIV infections and AIDS, but such a vaccine is probably years away from being available.

DYSLIPIDEMIA

Blood lipids are important risk factors for cardiovascular disease. A solid body of research, including animal, epidemiologic, and clinical studies, has established clearly that blood cholesterol, especially the subfraction low-density lipoprotein cholesterol (LDL-C), is a potent risk factor for development of CHD. It has also been convincingly demonstrated in several studies that lowering LDL levels with diet and drugs substantially lowers CVD rates. Clinical trial results have indicated that a 1% decrease in total or LDL-C will result in a 2% to 3% reduction in CHD rates. High-density lipoprotein cholesterol (HDL-C) is inversely related to CVD, and levels below 35 mg/dl are also considered a risk factor. Adult men in the United States have an average HDL-C level of 45 mg/dl compared to women with 55 mg/dl. This may partly explain why premenopausal women are at lower risk compared to men for development of CVD.

Dyslipidemia and high blood pressure are two conditions for which there is the most scientific evidence for treating and preventing cardiovascular disease.

Diet also plays an important role. A diet that is low in saturated fat and dietary cholesterol is complementary to weight loss and drugs for lowering LDL-C.

The National Heart, Lung and Blood Institute provides physicians with guidelines for managing blood lipids. These guidelines are provided in the second report of the National Cholesterol Education Program, Adult Treatment Panel. Table 9-6 summarizes these guidelines, which classify adult patients by presence of clinical disease, and presence or absence of CHD. In those patients without clinical CHD, total cholesterol and HDL-C levels are measured from a nonfasting blood sample. Subsequent fasting lipoproteins are then recommended in patients who have any of the following: (1) total cholesterol greater than or equal to 240 mg/dl, (2) HDL-C less than 35

TABLE 9-6.

Classification and Treatment Decisions Based on LDL Cholesterol[a]

Classification mg/dl
  < 130 Desirable LDL cholesterol
  130–159 Borderline high-risk LDL cholesterol
  ≥ 160 High-risk LDL cholesterol

	Initiation Level, mg/dl	Minimal Goal, mg/dl
Dietary treatment		
Without CHD or two other risk factors[b]	≥ 160	< 160[c]
With CHD or two other risk factors[b]	≥ 130	< 130[d]
Drug treatment		
Without CHD or two other risk factors[b]	≥ 190	< 160
With CHD or two other risk factors[b]	≥ 160	< 130

[a]LDL indicates low-density lipoprotein; CHD, coronary heart disease.

[b]Patients have a lower initiation level and goal if they are at high risk because they already have definite CHD, or because they have any two of the following risk factors: male sex, family history of premature CHD, cigarette smoking, hypertension, low high-density lipoprotein (HDL) cholesterol, diabetes mellitus, definite cerebrovascular or peripheral vascular disease, and severe obesity.

[c]Roughly equivalent to total cholesterol level of <240 mg/dl or <200 mg/dl.

[d]As goals for monitoring dietary treatment. Arch Intern Med 1988;148:36–69.

mg/dl, and (3) total cholesterol between 200 and 239 mg/dl and two or more other CHD risk factors. All patients with evidence of CHD should have fasting lipoproteins measured. Candidates for dietary advice are those with LDL-C level greater than or equal to 160 mg/dl or LDL-C level between 130 and 159 mg/dl in the presence of two or more risk factors. Those patients with clinical CHD should receive diet advice if their LDL-C level is greater than or equal to 100 mg/dl.

After dietary intervention, if plasma LDL-C levels remain at 30 mg/dl higher than baseline, then drug treatment should be considered. Patients with the following criteria would be eligible for drug treatment: (1) LDL-C level of 190 mg/dl or higher with no CHD and fewer than two CHD risk factors, (2) LDL-C level greater than or equal to 160 mg/dl for patients with two or more risk factors, or (3) LDL-C level greater than or equal to 130 mg/dl for patients with existing clinical CHD.

Using these criteria, approximately 40% of adults qualify for lipoprotein measurement, and almost 30% are in need of dietary therapy. A conservative estimate of adults who need drug therapy in addition to diet is 10% of adults in the United States. Hypolipidemic drugs include the HMG CoA reductase inhibitors (or the statins—lovastatin, pravastatin, and atorvastatin), resin-binding agents (e.g., cholestyramine), and fibric acid derivatives (e.g., gemfibrozil and nicotinic acid). It is currently possible to lower the level of LDL-C by 50% or more in many patients using diet and drug treatment. Figure 9-7 provides details on lipid management from the National Cholesterol Education Program, Adult Treatment Panel (panel III) guidelines.

SMOKING

Cigarette smoking causes much preventable illness and death and is, in fact, the **single most avoidable cause of death in the United States.** Cigarette smoking causes 85% of lung cancer cases in the United States and is linked substantially to cancer of the larynx, esophagus, mouth, pancreas, and bladder. Virtually all organs that come into direct or indirect contact with smoke or the metabolic byproducts have increased risk of cancer. It is the principal cause of chronic obstructive lung disease, and it has been estimated to **account for 25% of all**

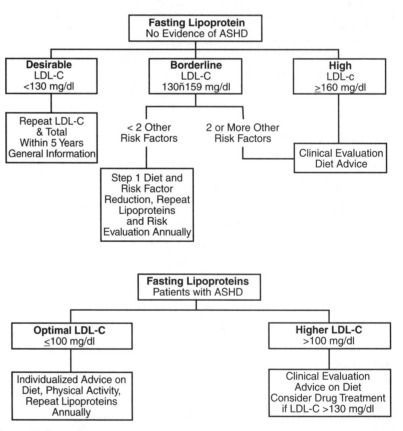

Figure 9-7.
Lipid management from the National Cholesterol Education Program, Adult Treatment Guidelines (panel III).

cardiovascular disease. In 1993, $50 billion in medical costs were attributed to cigarette smoking.

Smoking during pregnancy slows fetal growth and raises the risk of spontaneous abortion and fetal and neonatal death. The danger to health in persons living with smokers, by means of breathing passive smoke, is well established and has caused significant social concern. Smoking also contributes to accidental death and injury from fires and burns. Finally, the benefit of quitting smoking is clearly established; the overall mortality rate of ex-smokers after 15 years of cessation is similar to that of nonsmokers, and for cardiovascular disease, mortality rate is cut in half only 1 to 2 years after ceasing smoking.

More than 4000 specific substances have been identified in cigarette smoke. Most of these substances have not been studied and their health effects are unknown. Several are known to be pharmacologically active. Substances in smoke are divided into both gaseous and particulate matter. Carbon monoxide is the gas that causes the most concern. The particulate matter includes tar and is thought to be the cause of increased cancer risk associated with smoking. Objective measures of smoking are currently available and are in use in research studies. Cotinine and thiocyanate (a breakdown product of hydrogen cyanide) can be measured in the blood, urine, or saliva. Carbon monoxide exposure can be measured by carboxyhemoglobin study or in expired carbon monoxide.

Smoking, especially cigarettes, can be viewed as a highly efficient way to deliver the drug nicotine into the body. Nicotine, a toxic alkaloid, is highly addictive and has numerous adverse metabolic effects, including vasoconstriction with acute increases in blood pressure, myocardial oxygen consumption, cardiac arrhythmias, and increased force of myocardial contraction. This leads to increased myocardial oxygen consumption, which can precipitate angina pectoris or acute myocardial infarction in susceptible patients. Cigarette smokers overall have lower levels of HDL-C compared to nonsmokers. A lower level of HDL-C is a major risk factor for cardiovascular disease. Effects on HDL-C have been postulated to be one mechanism of how smoking causes CHD.

It has become apparent that "sidestream," or passive, smoke also represents significant risk for the same conditions. This concern over passive smoke has led to increased legislative action to ban or limit smoking in public areas in many states.

Even in the face of these known health hazards, many smokers find it difficult to give up this powerful addiction. Key strategies in the cessation of smoking include facilitating the individual's decision to quit, using a self-guided cessation program, or participating in an organized group program with social support. Cessation methods have included behavior modification, aversive conditioning, biofeedback, hypnosis, acupuncture, and nicotine replacement. Smoking cessation efforts in the United States have been very successful. Many adults have successfully quit smoking using these methods. About half of middle-aged men who ever smoked have quit; and currently only approximately 23% of US adults smoke. Likelihood of success in quitting is related to how heavily a person smokes. Using the statistics of total smoking-attributable deaths and years of potential life lost, smoking in the United States continues to be a major contributor to death and disability, even though smoking rates have declined. African Americans have a higher smoking-attributable mortality rate and years of potential life lost compared to whites. The prevention of smoking in young people is also very important in advancing public health. Recent trends show alarming increases in smoking rates among US teenagers, especially African American teenagers, since 1992. In the late 1990s, lung cancer deaths were decreasing in men but increasing in women; in 1987, **lung cancer deaths surpassed breast cancer as the number one cause of cancer deaths in women.** These trends can be attributed to smoking rate declines in men and increases in women over the past 30 years. National efforts are under way to prohibit or limit smoking in public places, and most states have passed aggressive antismoking legislation and are currently working to prohibit sales of cigarettes to minors. Other efforts include banning cigarette advertising directed at youth and restricting sale of cigarettes to minors through the use of heavy penalties and aggressive enforcement strategies. Recently, several states (e.g., Minnesota and Florida) and health care groups have sued the tobacco industry to recover health-related costs. Proceeds from these suits will be invested in smoking-related research.

Smoking cessation is clearly beneficial in reducing risk, especially for cardiovascular disease. In the Multiple Risk Factor Intervention Trial, middle-aged men who quit smoking experienced a 50% lower rate of subsequent CHD events compared to nonquitters. This benefit was seen as early as 1 year after quitting. Other studies have suggested that risk for lung cancer is partially reduced by quitting smoking. However, if this occurs, it is over a much longer period of time, 10 years or more.

OBESITY

Obesity is a colossal health problem in the United States. The NHANES III conducted in the mid-1990s found that one third of US adults are overweight, roughly 58 million Americans. Obesity is an epidemic in the United States; it is by far the most common nutritional disorder. Obesity is associated with higher risk of mortality from a number of diseases, including artherosclerotic heart disease, stroke, and diabetes mellitus. Blood pressure and blood lipid levels are strongly related to obesity.

Body weight increases with age. In men, the highest rate of obesity occurs at ages 50 to 69 years (42%) and in women at ages 50 to 59 years (52%).

Americans have been gaining weight at alarming rates (Table 9-7). Since 1975, obesity (and diabetes) are the only major CHD risk

TABLE 9-7.		
NHANES Prevalence of Overweight by Percent		

Group	1976 – 1980	1988 – 1991
All adults		
Ages 20 – 74	25.4	33.3
White		
Men	24.2	32.0
Women	44.5	49.2
African American		
Men	26.2	31.8
Women	44.5	49.2

factors that have increased. High blood pressure, abnormal blood lipid levels, and cigarette smoking have all decreased in prevalence over the same time period.

Obesity is even more prevalent among certain ethnic groups. **African-American women have the highest prevalence (48.6%),** but obesity is also a problem in Mexican-American women (46.7%) and white women (32.9%).

Overweight prevalence in men is lower than in women, but it is still unacceptably high: Mexican-American men (35.5%), white men (32.3%), and African-American men (30.9%) (Figure 9-8).

The trend of increased obesity in the US population continues to

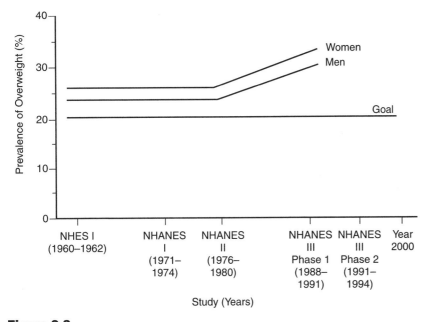

Figure 9-8.
Trends in age-adjusted prevalence of overweight for persons 20 through 74 years of age in the United States, compared with the year 2000 health objective for overweight. NHES, National Health Examination Survey; NHANES, National Health and Nutrition Examination Survey.

increase. Between the NHANES II survey in 1976 to 1980 and the NHANES III (1988 to 1991), the prevalence of overweight adults increased from 25.4% to 33.3% or, on average, about an 8-pound increase.

The causes of this marked increase are not known, but lack of and reduced physical activity is considered a major suspect; 58% of US adults report either inadequate or irregular leisure time activity.

Because obesity is so strongly related to high blood pressure, abnormal lipid levels, and diabetes, it will be an increasing public health priority in the future to try to control the epidemic. In June 1998, the National Heart, Lung and Blood Institute and the National Institute of Diabetes, Digestive and Kidney Diseases published the first National Institutes of Health (NIH) guidelines on obesity for medical practitioners called the "Clinical Guidelines on the Identification, Evaluation and Treatment of Overweight and Obese Adults." The report stated that obesity is second only to cigarette smoking as the most preventable cause of death in the United States.

These guidelines are patterned after previous NIH guidelines on high blood pressure and blood cholesterol. Obesity is best defined in terms of body mass index, or **BMI,** which is body weight measured in kilograms divided by height in centimeters squared (BMI = weight [kg]/height^2 [cm^2]). Obesity is defined as a BMI greater than or equal to 30, and overweight is 25 kg/m^2 or more. Using this definition, almost 100 million Americans are overweight or obese. The report states that BMI should be measured in all patients and reassessed at least **every 2 years.**

The best measure for **central obesity** according to the guidelines is waist circumference, which is preferred over the commonly used waist-to-hip ratio. In people with BMI in the 23.5 to 34.9 range, a waist circumference of more than 40 inches in men and of more than 35 inches in women represents significant risk.

The guidelines call for lifestyle intervention for at least 6 months before considering drug therapy. Drug therapy (for up to 1 year) may be tried in high-risk obese patients, that is, in patients whose BMI is greater than or equal to 30 regardless of risk factors or greater than or equal to 27 with at least two major risk factors. **Risk factors** include diabetes mellitus, high blood pressure, hyperlipidemia, and sleep apnea.

PHYSICAL ACTIVITY

Physical fitness relates significantly to the ability of one to effectively perform work, household chores, sports, and dance. Only 40% of American adults regularly exercise. Physical activity is recommended at least 3 days a week, lasting at least 20 minutes a session. The sessions should be sufficiently intense to use a minimum of 300 kcal and must be continued regularly to maintain a training effect.

The time that adults spend on vigorous activity has increased since the 1970s. It seems likely, however, that an individual commitment to improve physical fitness is needed to spur this activity. Certain demographic groups, including women, older adults, inner city residents, rural residents, and persons from low-income groups, show low participation in exercise and should be particularly encouraged by physicians to take advantage of its benefits.

The rhythmic use of large muscle groups does reduce the risk of coronary heart disease and slows the loss of calcium in postmenopausal women. Physical activity also modestly helps in controlling hypertension, improves lipid profile, and increases the effect of insulin in patients with insulin-dependent diabetes mellitus. The antidepressant effect of exercise is well known. Long-term studies have strongly suggested that regular sustained physical activity consisting of 2000 kcal of energy expenditure per week will help prevent cardiovascular disease. This is a level comparable to walking 3 miles a day.

ALCOHOL

Misuse of alcohol and other drugs is a worldwide health hazard. Both the toxic effect and the increased risk of injury and death while under their influence constitute the medical consequences. The personal, family, social, and occupational effects of alcohol and drug addiction are disastrous. Other less commonly abused drugs include illicit drugs such as marijuana, heroin, and cocaine, and legal drugs used for nonmedical purposes. Tranquilizers, barbiturates, and amphetamines have been among the most abused prescription drugs. The effect sought is primarily a dulling of normal emotional feelings and appropriate processing of those feelings.

Regulatory measures have been the nation's primary tool to reduce these problems. For example, US **federal legislation has sought to induce states to adopt 21 years of age as the minimum age for drinking alcohol;** such legislation restricts a portion of highway construction funds until the state has passed the desired laws. Educational programs have also been tried, including special information programs for high-risk populations, including physicians themselves. In one national program, hospital emergency departments report admissions for abuse. In recent years, alcohol combined with other drugs has been a leading cause of both admissions and deaths in emergency departments. Alcohol and drug abuse is also a major risk among physicians and health care workers. This is in part due to easier access to drugs. Treatment programs with good success rates based on the "12-step" program are widely available. Identification of the addiction problem by the patient, family, and friends, and active involvement in treatment are essential to controlling this progressive disease. Successful treatment programs involve the entire family and employers in the treatment process.

Alcoholism and drug addiction are highly prevalent health problems. Approximately 90% of US adults consume alcohol and, overall, at least 10% of men and 5% of women are alcoholics. Alcoholism is prominent in all levels of society, in all ethnic groups, income groups, and education groups. For alcoholics, alcohol intake is a compulsion and has major life-limiting effects. Alcoholism significantly affects all areas of life—personal, family, social, and occupational. It is a major cause of violence and accidents. The American Psychiatric Association separates patients with alcohol problems into two main categories: (1) those who abuse alcohol, for whom alcohol intake impairs life functioning and (2) those whose problems consist of alcohol dependence-impaired life functioning combined with a compulsion for alcohol. Alcohol dependence over time is usually associated with the development of increased tolerance and, when intake is stopped, withdrawal symptoms. Alcohol dependence is a progressive disease, which, if not successfully treated, will kill or disable the patient.

In clinical practice, significant alcoholism can be identified by the following consequences: (1) marital separation or divorce; (2) loss of employment; (3) arrests for alcohol-related charges, such as driving while intoxicated, and (4) alcohol-related health problems (e.g., cirrhosis, esophageal varices, cardiomyopathy).

Pregnant women who drink any amount of alcohol are at risk for complications of pregnancy, including spontaneous abortions. Children born to women who drink during pregnancy are at high risk for fetal alcohol syndrome or the more prevalent fetal alcohol effect. Both are accompanied by mental retardation. These conditions are frequently also associated with extreme behavior problems, including lack of judgment. Ironically, fetal alcohol conditions are totally preventable, if the mother is not exposed to alcohol during the pregnancy. Risk of fetal effects is present even at low levels of intake, so the recommendation to the patient is to not consume alcohol at all during pregnancy.

Because of the dire social and health effects of alcohol dependence, physicians should be alert to diagnosing an alcohol problem. A frequently used screening questionnaire is called the Michigan Alcohol Screening Test (MAST). Most alcoholics will not admit they have a problem and will not seek care on their own.

Once a diagnosis of alcoholism is made, it is important to involve the family and confront the alcohol problem in a controlled way. It is important to involve other significant family and friends and, with a unified group, confront the patient with his or her problem. This process is termed "an intervention."

Most communities have alcohol and drug addiction treatment resources. Most of the programs are based on the "12-step" model, which has a respectable track record of success. Alcoholics Anonymous (AA) is available for aftercare.

Support for the family of the addict is important also, and resources such as Alanon and Alateen are available for family members. These teach the family members how to avoid supporting the affected family member's addiction. Once treatment has been initiated, ideally it should last for at least 6 to 12 months.

Among other major additional addictive illegal drugs are cocaine, heroin, and methamphetamines. Prescription drugs that are commonly abused include tranquilizers, barbiturates, amphetamines, and pain medication. Because physicians, nurses, pharmacists, and other health care workers have relatively easy access to drugs, they are at higher risk for drug abuse. Another especially high-risk group is patients with chronic pain syndrome who abuse analgesics. Treatment approaches to drug addiction use similar methods and interventions as for alcoholism. This approach is also used for treating other forms of addictions, such as chronic gambling.

NUTRITION

In recent years, the focus of nutritional science has moved from curing deficiency diseases to searching for relationships between diet and chronic disease and to investigating the role of diet in promoting health. Increased public awareness about these relationships causes patients to ask for sophisticated nutritional advice from their personal physicians. In the United States, the population has decreased its intake of fat, whole milk, eggs, beef, and pork. Many patients seek the advice of their physicians in their attempts to improve their diets. Physicians can help by reinforcing positive changes and by making referrals to community resources such as nutritionists.

OLDER ADULTS

Achievements in disease prevention and treatment in recent decades have increased the life expectancy of many adults who would formerly have died of heart disease, stroke, cancer, or other major causes of death. The expanding survival rate has changed the nation's demography. The proportion of the population aged 65 years and older has increased markedly. Among that group, those aged 85 and older form the fastest growing segment of the population (Table 9-8). Life expectancy has increased less for men than for women, who form an increasing majority of older age groups, so much so that discussants commonly infer that the problem of aging is particularly a problem of women. These changes by gender have had significant implications for the economics and health of the United States, and the expanding survival rate generally has influenced many political decisions about organizing and financing contemporary health care in the United States.

In the 1980s, the population of persons aged 65 years and older formed 12% of the total population, with approximately 150 women

TABLE 9-8.

Changing Age Distribution of the Older Population (United States, 1950–2020)

	Percent 65–69 years	Percent 70–84 years	Percent 85+ years	Ratio $\dfrac{65\text{–}69}{85+}$
1950	41	55	5	9
1960	38	57	6	7
1970	35	58	7	5
1980	34	57	9	4
1990	32	58	11	3
2000	26	59	15	2
2010	30	53	17	2
2020	32	53	14	2

U.S. Bureau of the Census, 1984, "Demographic and Socioeconomic Aspects of Aging in the United States," Current Population Reports, *Series P-23, No. 138.*

Over time, the older population of the United States will itself be growing older (that is, higher percentages aged 85+), at least until the "Baby Boom" generation reaches old age.

for every 100 men. Proportionately more men have a spouse living. Thus, men are more often cared for at home and less often admitted to nursing homes. At any one time, approximately 5% of those aged 65 years and older are in nursing homes, with most residents being women. Approximately 30% of older adults live alone and have little opportunity to discuss their health problems with a family member. Such persons become more dependent on their family physician for advice and help. Visiting nurses who deliver care in homes find that most of their clients are women; when called to help a disabled man living with his spouse at home, the nurse usually finds a more severely disabled male who has been able to stay at home because of the physical help given by his spouse. Thus, the demography of elderly persons plays an important role in health care needs.

In both sexes of older adults, the major causes of death have decreased. Diseases of the heart and cerebrovascular diseases have decreased substantially in recent decades, probably because of better lifestyles and detection. In contrast, cancers have not changed much, partly because of an increase in lung cancer in women who have increased their cigarette exposure in recent decades.

Among elderly adults, the causes of impaired function differ from causes of death. Thus, the arthritides affect 44% of persons aged 65 years and older, with women being more often and more seriously impaired than men of the same age. While rarely causing hospital admission, arthritis is the cause of many visits to physicians and approximately 16% of all disability days spent in bed. Deafness and impaired visual acuity are also major losses of function; they diminish quality of life but rarely cause death.

Older persons smoke less than persons in younger age groups because cigarette smokers are less likely to survive into old age and because smokers tend to quit as they age. Of the 16% who do smoke, there is good evidence that health improves after quitting. Older persons tend to exercise less regularly than younger groups. Scalding from hot water is the leading cause of burns in elderly persons. Osteoporosis and easily fractured hips are potential causes of impairment and death; the prominence of these causes will be lessened in elderly women in the coming decades as improvements in nutrition are made and as effective new pharmacologic and surgical treatment modalities become available.

Even at a late age in older patients, behavior may be changed to improve health and alleviate discomfort. Prevention efforts are not wasted on older patients.

FAMILY PLANNING

Family planning is based on the voluntary decisions and actions of individuals who want to reduce unintended fertility or to correct infertility. This effort may or may not be compatible with national population policy, but it helps individuals and couples decide for themselves about reproduction. In recent decades in the United States, patterns have changed, and many women are waiting until their 30s and 40s to begin families. In addition, more single women are having children. Family size has decreased as women have fewer children and fertility rates decline.

Sterilization has become more common among married women. Oral contraceptives remain popular with unmarried women, as does the use of condoms by unmarried men. Teenagers exhibit high rates of unintended pregnancy, abortion, and low use of contraceptive methods. Teenage pregnancies are associated with increased risks of maternal morbidity and mortality. Thus, teenagers who are sexually active are a prime target for birth control efforts.

On the other hand, millions of couples are infertile, unable, or unlikely to have children. One fourth of these couples are childless. Proportionately more African American than white couples are infertile. The technology for improving fertility rates is rapidly advancing, for example, through in vitro fertilization and surrogate births. Gene technology will soon have a significant impact on the field, and spiritual and ethical issues have been raised. It will be a challenge for the pace of societal ethics to keep up with this rapidly developing technology. Private medical sources provide most access to infertility care in the United States where African Americans and other minorities often lack access to this form of care. Policy debates have usually focused on the ethics and financing of abortion and less on family planning.

PREGNANCY AND INFANT HEALTH

Since 1960, maternal and infant death rates have declined steadily in the United States. The rate of decline was 5% to 6% per year in the 1970s but less than 3% per year in the 1990s. African American and unmarried mothers account for a proportionately high percentage of low-birth-weight infants, who sustain higher-than-average infant mortality rates despite costly improvements in neonatal intensive care. African-American infant mortality rates are nearly double those of whites. A recent development that impairs access to quality care for all patients is the tendency of physicians and hospitals to withdraw from high-risk obstetric care for marketplace and malpractice reasons.

The success of programs for pregnancy and infant health depends partly on other health programs, such as programs for environmental control, nutrition, and communicable disease. Mortality and morbidity rates range markedly between different population groups and geographic regions. Cigarette smoking during pregnancy is associated with birth weights that are 150 g to 200 g lower than average. Maternal alcohol intake during pregnancy is one of the most common causes of mental retardation. Untreated diabetes in mothers is a potent risk factor for congenital anomalies in infants. Congenital anomalies, the highest cause of infant death, are equally common in African American and white infants (Table 9-9). Most other causes of infant death, such as the respiratory distress syndrome and infections, are more common in African Americans. The newborns are commonly screened in hospitals for the **early detection of phenylketonuria (PKU) and hypothyroidism.**

TABLE 9-9.

Top 10 Causes of Infant Mortality by Race, United States, 1983 (Deaths per 100,000 Live Births)

Rank	Cause	All	Race African American	White
1	Congenital anomalies	240.0	246.2	241.9
2	Sudden infant death syndrome	145.8	259.0	124.4
3	Respiratory distress syndrome	101.2	159.4	92.1
4	Disorders related to short gestation and low birth weight	91.6	228.3	66.5
5	Maternal complication	39.9	73.7	34.4
6	Intrauterine hypoxia and birth asphyxia	32.9	56.0	29.1
7	Accidents and adverse effects	26.3	45.6	23.0
8	Infections specific to the perinatal period	23.9	36.7	21.7
9	Newborn affected by complications of placenta, cord, and membranes	23.9	16.9	11.6
10	Pneumonia and influenza	21.1	47.6	16.0

Breast feeding has been shown to prevent both malnutrition and obesity in infants. Moreover, it may provide the infant with short-term immunity from some infectious diseases. The number of women who breast fed their infants more than doubled to 53% by 1980, increasing more swiftly in white mothers than in African American mothers. On the more technical side, diagnostic ultrasound has become more frequent in obstetrics, and electronic fetal monitoring is used on half or more mothers in labor. Rates of cesarean section deliveries have been increasing. It is unclear how many of these high-tech and surgical approaches are medically indicated and how many are carried out because of malpractice concerns, economic reasons, and convenience. High-quality and readily accessible prenatal care can decrease the risk of low birth weight and other complications.

GENETIC SCREENING

The capacity for genetic screening for inherited disorders has grown exponentially since 1990. Screening for birth defects begins in the fetal period when women are offered tests for prenatal diagnosis. All women are offered screening tests for neural tube defects by maternal serum alpha-fetoprotein (AFP). An **elevated AFP is associated with an open neural defect. A low AFP has been found to be associated with trisomy 21 (Down syndrome).** Screening for trisomy 21 is also offered to women of advanced maternal age, 35 years or older. There is specialized testing done for families who have already had an affected child with a genetic disorder such as cystic fibrosis or who are at risk based on ethnic background. The majority of screening is done by amniocentesis routinely offered between 15 and 20 weeks' gestation. Some perinatal centers also offer **chorionic villus sampling,** which can be done at an earlier gestational age, somewhere between 10 and 11 weeks of gestation.

Newborn screening is routinely performed in all 50 states. Screening is focused on disorders that are life threatening if early intervention is missed or where early intervention prevents profound mental retardation. All states screen for congenital hypothyroidism and PKU. In addition, the majority of states screen for hemoglobinopathies and galactosemia. Several states screen for congenital adrenal hyperplasia and cystic fibrosis.

Susceptibility screening for adult disorders is a rapidly growing field. Currently, testing is available for some cancer syndromes such as breast cancer or colon cancer. Testing for other late-onset disorders, such as cardiovascular disease, may become available in the future. The management of screening individuals from a fetus to an adult has become a complex process. The screening needs to be accompanied by appropriate genetic counseling before testing as well as when test results become available.

COMMUNITY HEALTH QUESTIONS

<hr />

MULTIPLE CHOICE QUESTIONS

Choose the BEST answer for each question. Answers are at the end of this chapter.

1. Efforts to support the use of lifestyle changes (e.g., weight loss, reduction in dietary saturated fat) across the entire community

    (A) are not useful because only a few people will make significant lifestyle changes
    (B) are useful in preventing disease even if only small mean changes in risk factors occur in the population
    (C) are not worthwhile because even if lifestyle changes are made they cannot be maintained
    (D) should be mainly based using the medical model in physician office practices
    (E) A and C above

2. The "population perspective" refers to the following:

    (A) Risk factors in one population cannot be extrapolated to another
    (B) It is only useful from a public health perspective
    (C) The disease will best be prevented by focusing on higher risk patients
    (D) Minor changes in the average level of the risk factors in the population are best in preventing the total number of people getting clinical disease

3. Reduction of blood cholesterol in the population achieved through dietary changes and weight loss would result in the largest amount of heart disease prevented in which of the following groups?

(A) Hypercholesterolemic patients
(B) People with above average to "high normal" to "mild elevations" in blood cholesterol
(C) Patients with BMI greater than or equal to 30 kg/m²
(D) Patients with BMI greater than or equal to 27 and LDL-C greater than or equal to 190 mg/dl

4. Who is responsible for filling out the death certificate?

(A) Attending physician
(B) Chief of staff
(C) Funeral director
(D) Nurses
(E) None of the above

5. Whose job is it to file the birth certificate with the registrar after a delivery?

(A) Nurse coordinator
(B) The hospital where delivery occurred
(C) Nurse
(D) Attending physician
(E) None of the above

6. Who has the final responsibility for assigning cause of death on the death certificate?

(A) Physician
(B) Nosologist
(C) Senior resident
(D) Nurse
(E) None of the above

7. Which of the following factors influences crude death rates?

(A) Age
(B) Gender
(C) Ethnicity
(D) Marital status
(E) All of the above

8. The highest prevalence of obesity is in which ethnic group?

   (A) African-American women
   (B) African-American men
   (C) White women
   (D) Mexican-American men

9. Between the NHANES II (1976 to 1980) and the NHANES III (1988 to 1991) studies, what has been the average amount of weight gained in the American adult?

   (A) 3 lb
   (B) 5 lb
   (C) 2 lb
   (D) 8 lb
   (E) 0 lb

10. Which of the following explanations is likely an important cause of increasing obesity in the United States?

    (A) Increased carbohydrates in the diet
    (B) Heredity
    (C) Irregular and inadequate levels of physical activity
    (D) Increased fat in diet as a percent of calories

11. Three standard deviations (SD) on both sides of the mean in a normal distribution encompass which percent of the data?

    (A) 99.7%
    (B) 95.4%
    (C) 75.1%
    (D) 68.3%
    (E) 34.1%

12. What is another term for a "normal distribution?"

    (A) Pearson
    (B) Gaussian
    (C) Student's t
    (D) Cox
    (E) ANOVA

13. According to a 1998 report by the National Heart, Lung and Blood Institute and the National Institute of Diabetes, Digestive and Kidney Diseases, approximately how many US adults are overweight or obese?

(A) More than 200 million
(B) Almost 100 million
(C) 50 million
(D) 25 million

14. Which measure is considered the best measure of central obesity?

(A) Waist-to-hip ratio
(B) Hip circumference
(C) Chest circumference
(D) Waist circumference

15. According to NIH guidelines on overweight and obesity, what is the preferred measure for defining obesity?

(A) Body weight in kilograms
(B) Body surface area (BSA)
(C) Waist-to-hip ratio
(D) Body mass index (BMI)

16. According to NIH guidelines, how often should patients be assessed for overweight or obesity in medical practice?

(A) Every 6 months
(B) Every year
(C) Every 2 years
(D) Every 5 years
(E) As needed

17. After 6 months of lifestyle intervention, National Institutes of Health guidelines state that drug treatment can be considered in high-risk obese patients. How is high risk defined?

(A) BMI greater than or equal to 35
(B) BMI 23.5 to 27 with at least two risk factors
(C) BMI greater than or equal to 30 regardless of risk factors
(D) None of the above

18. What are the risk factors that are listed when deciding to use drug treatment for obesity?

(A) Diabetes
(B) High blood pressure
(C) High cholesterol level
(D) Sleep apnea
(E) All of the above

19. Which of the following statements is correct concerning case-control studies?

(A) Observed associations cannot establish causation
(B) Case-control studies cannot raise important clinical questions
(C) Case-control studies are cheaper and superior to trials for evaluating treatments
(D) Case-control studies are no more likely to be subject to treatment selection bias than are clinical trials

20. What is a good way to reduce or eliminate endpoint ascertainment bias in a clinical trial?

(A) Carefully define the clinical endpoints
(B) Standardize measurement procedures
(C) Control for frequency of contact
(D) Ensure that the ascertainment observers are blinded to study groups
(E) All of the above

21. A study was reported comparing a new antibiotic to penicillin for relapse rates of pneumococcal pneumonia. It was a parallel double-blind study treating cases and following up patients for 6 months. Thirty patients were randomized to two groups, with 15 in each group. The study results showed a relapse rate of 15% with penicillin and 22% with the new drug. The P value on this difference was 0.35. What is the most likely explanation of this result?

(A) The new antibiotic is superior to penicillin
(B) The study made a type I error
(C) There is no difference between the two antibiotics
(D) The study lacks statistical power
(E) The study design was flawed

22. The "power" in a study is best defined as

(A) having an insufficient sample size
(B) chances of not making a type II error
(C) alpha error
(D) chances of making a type I error
(E) none of the above

23. A large health maintenance organization retrospective data set analysis shows that patients given diuretics are *more* likely to die of heart failure. This is a surprise because diuretics are one of the treatments for heart failure. What is the most likely explanation of this result?

(A) Treatment selection bias
(B) Diuretics are harmful
(C) Diagnosis of heart failure in the data is unreliable
(D) Endpoint ascertainment bias

24. What is the main reason to use "double-blind" methods in a study?

(A) Reduce endpoint ascertainment bias
(B) Minimize patients going off drug
(C) Increase study credibility
(D) Reduce observer measurement bias

25. The "placebo effect" observed in many studies can frequently be explained by

(A) faulty study design
(B) regression to the mean
(C) unknown biologic effects to placebo
(D) observer measurement bias

26. When used alone, the statin drugs for lowering cholesterol (lovastatin, pravastatin, and atorvastatin) would be expected to reduce LDL-C by what magnitude in most patients?

(A) 10%
(B) 80%
(C) 20% to 40%
(D) 10% to 25%

27. A 15% reduction in total and LDL-C would be estimated to reduce CHD risk by what degree?

    (A) 30% to 45%
    (B) 5% to 15%
    (C) 100%
    (D) 5% to 10%
    (E) 0% to 5%

28. What is the single most avoidable factor responsible for deaths in the United States?

    (A) Cigarette smoking
    (B) Diabetes mellitus
    (C) End-stage renal disease
    (D) Dyslipidemia
    (E) Depression

29. Which of the following diseases became the number one cause of death from cancer in women after 1987?

    (A) Lung cancer
    (B) Ovarian cancer
    (C) Uterine cancer
    (D) Colon cancer
    (E) Brain cancer

30. Clinical trial evidence suggests that, by quitting smoking, death from cardiovascular disease can be reduced by approximately 50% by what time period?

    (A) 5 years
    (B) 0 years
    (C) 20 years
    (D) As early as 1 year

31. Likelihood of quitting smoking is most strongly related to

    (A) physician advice to quit
    (B) number of cigarettes smoked per day
    (C) history of quit attempts
    (D) spouse support

32. What is the proportion of all cardiovascular disease in the United States that is attributed to cigarette smoking?

(A) 25%
(B) 50%
(C) 55%
(D) 5%
(E) 10%

33. Over recent years, which ethnic subgroup of adolescents has experienced the largest increase in smoking rates?

(A) African Americans
(B) Whites
(C) Asian Americans
(D) Mexican Americans
(E) Cuban Americans

34. Over what time period was the NHANES III phase 2 survey conducted?

(A) 1991 to 1994
(B) 1975 to 1979
(C) 1979 to 1982
(D) 1989 to 1991

35. What regular publication from the Centers for Disease Control updates physicians on recent issues and recommendations on public health?

(A) *The Medical Letter*
(B) The Surgeon General's Report
(C) *HLB Newsletter*
(D) *Mortality and Morbidity Weekly Report* (MMWR)

36. Rates of obesity in women and girls in the United States are highest in which ethnic subgroup?

(A) African American, non-Hispanic
(B) Mexican American
(C) White non-Hispanic
(D) Asian, Pacific Islanders

37. Case-control studies in postmenopausal women have observed that women taking estrogen hormone replacement therapy (HRT) are about half as likely to have coronary heart disease (CHD) compared to non-users. What are reasonable interpretations of these findings?

    (A) HRT may prevent CHD
    (B) Women HRT-users may be in many ways more health conscious than non-users
    (C) HRT use may be related to socioeconomic status
    (D) All of the above

38. What are the limitations of treatments derived from animal models and mechanistic pathways?

    (A) Animal models are rarely directly extrapolated to humans
    (B) Related but important physiologic and biochemical mechanisms are unknown
    (C) Clinical trials conducted later frequently do not provide validation
    (D) All of the above

39. The best information for basing medical treatment recommendations comes from

    (A) Meta-analysis
    (B) A single, large, well-designed, sufficiently powered clinical trial
    (C) Journal review articles
    (D) Clinical judgment
    (E) *The Wall Street Journal*

40. How are study dropouts likely to be different from trial participants?

    (A) Smoking prevalence
    (B) Adherence to study drug
    (C) Endpoint event rates
    (D) All of the above
    (E) None of the above

41. Since the mid-1970s, prevalence of obesity in the United States has increased substantially in which group?

    (A) Women
    (B) People 60 years of age and older
    (C) African Americans
    (D) White, non-Hispanics
    (E) All of the above

42. A managed-care data set shows that cardiovascular disease was more likely to develop in patients given calcium channel blockers compared to patients given diuretics. The classic problem of inability to separate cause versus effect is inherent using which study method?

    (A) Case-control study
    (B) Observational study
    (C) Clinical trial
    (D) Case reports

43. Which of the following is the largest single cause of maternal mortality?

    (A) Toxemia (hypertensive disease) of pregnancy
    (B) Ectopic pregnancies
    (C) Poor prenatal care
    (D) Breech deliveries
    (E) Preterm abortions

44. Another term for a type II error is

    (A) Sigma error
    (B) Pearson error
    (C) Alpha error
    (D) Beta error
    (E) None of the above

45. What was the main contributing factor for the marked increase in life expectancy from birth observed from around 1910 to 1950?

    (A) Increased physical activity
    (B) Low rates of cigarette smoking
    (C) Control of common childhood infectious diseases
    (D) Good nutrition
    (E) Penicillin

46. What official group in the United States established and updated guidelines for diagnosing, treating, and preventing high blood pressure?

(A) Joint National Committee (JNC)
(B) World Health Organization (WHO)
(C) American Society of Hypertension (ASH)
(D) American College of Physicians (ACP)
(E) None of the above

47. What percent of hypertensives in the United States had adequately controlled blood pressure in the mid-1990s?

(A) 58%
(B) 38%
(C) 27%
(D) 20%
(E) 88%

48. What best describes the mortality rate from stroke in the United States from the 1920s to the late 1990s?

(A) Continues to decline sharply
(B) Continues to decline but at a slower rate
(C) Has leveled off
(D) Has leveled off and is increasing substantially
(E) Has increased substantially

49. What percent of hypertensives was aware of their condition in the mid-1990s?

(A) 33%
(B) 25%
(C) 68%
(D) 73%
(E) 76%

50. What percent of hypertensives was treated with drugs in the NHANES III phase II survey carried out in 1991 to 1994?

(A) 53%
(B) 10%
(C) 68%
(D) 25%
(E) None of the above

51. According to the JNC VI guidelines, drug treatment should be used initially in patients with high normal blood pressures (systolic blood pressure 130 to 139 mm Hg or diastolic blood pressure 85 to 89 mm Hg) under which of the following circumstances?

   (A) The patient has more than three cardiovascular risk factors
   (B) The patient has diabetes mellitus
   (C) The patient has failed on 3 months of lifestyle treatment
   (D) The patient has hyperlipidemia
   (E) None of the above

52. Which of the following are not recommended by JNC VI as preventive or adjunctive lifestyle treatments for high blood pressure?

   (A) Relaxation and meditation
   (B) Weight loss
   (C) Dietary sodium reduction
   (D) Increased physical activity
   (E) Reduced alcohol intake if moderate or heavy drinker

53. What is the most important consideration in the initial prescribing of thiazide diuretics in patients with uncomplicated hypertension?

   (A) Use only with potassium sparing agents
   (B) Increase dose until desired blood pressure response is obtained
   (C) Avoid using because of adverse metabolic effects
   (D) Use low dose that is primarily up to 25 mg daily of hydrochlorothiazide or chlorthalidone or equivalent doses of other thiazides
   (E) None of the above

54. Which of the following was emphasized by JNC VI for the control of high blood pressure?

   (A) Start drugs at low dose and titrate slowly
   (B) Use multiple drugs when initiating blood pressure treatments
   (C) Use drugs with long duration of action
   (D) Increase use of combination drug therapy
   (E) All of the above

55. What type of blood pressure drugs in addition to diuretic has been shown to reduce stroke in a major clinical trial (Systolic Hypertension Studies in Europe)?

(A) Angiotensin receptor blockers
(B) Alpha-beta blockers
(C) Alpha blockers
(D) Loop diuretics
(E) Long-acting dihydropyridine calcium blockers

56. The ultimate public health goal of preventing high blood pressure is

(A) 90% to 100% treatment and control
(B) 80% to 100% adherence to medical therapy
(C) prevention of hypertension by improving relevant lifestyles in the population
(D) coordination of blood pressure management with treating other cardiovascular disease risk factors

57. A small (n = 30) double-blind clinical trial comparing a new drug treatment to placebo for relief of dysmenorrhea shows a 50% reduction in pain symptoms using the new drug versus a placebo control. The P value of this difference is 0.01. Which of these statements is correct?

(A) The study is too small and has insufficient power
(B) Placebo is not the most appropriate control in this study
(C) The study by definition has sufficient power
(D) It was unethical to use placebo in this study
(E) All of the above

58. A risk factor is defined as

(A) a modifiable factor, which, if changed, will reduce the chances of disease
(B) a factor that causes the disease
(C) a continuous variable that is sometimes associated with increased risk
(D) a factor that, if present, gives an individual a higher probability of acquiring the disease

59. What is the definition of an *independent* risk factor?

    (A) A factor that places an individual at increased risk and cannot be accounted for by a relationship to other factors

    (B) A factor that is strongly related to chances of developing a disease

    (C) A factor that is associated with risk and is modifiable

    (D) A factor that is specific for the disease

60. A large study is conducted comparing two antihypertensive drugs (diuretic versus beta blocker) for lowering cardiovascular mortality and morbidity. At the end of 5 years, the study dropout rate is 20% in the diuretic group and 10% with the beta blocker. What is the most serious concern with the study data?

    (A) Generalization of the study results

    (B) High dropout rates invalidate the study results

    (C) In the analysis, results should be adjusted for the different dropout rates

    (D) The dropout rate is different between treatment groups

61. What action would best address this dropout problem?

    (A) Put efforts into lowering the dropout rates in both study groups

    (B) Adjust data for differential dropout rates

    (C) Limit the analysis to only study patients who did not drop out

    (D) Invalidate study results

    (E) Recruit more patients into both groups

62. What is the best method for ensuring that patients assigned to different study groups are similar in severity of disease at entry?

    (A) Blocking treatment assignments

    (B) Extensive baseline medical evaluations

    (C) Randomization

    (D) Adjusting entry criteria

    (E) All of the above

63. The main emphasis in managed care is to accomplish the following:

   (A) Improve quality of health care delivered
   (B) Organize means to provide acceptable quality of care with reduced costs
   (C) Improve patient-physician communication
   (D) Prevent acute and chronic diseases

64. Future challenges for managed care include

   (A) Assessing quality (effectiveness) of new and existing treatments
   (B) Controlling costs in an increasing environment of new drugs and devices
   (C) Accommodating education, training, and research within their mission
   (D) Increasing focus on prevention
   (E) All of the above

65. The main methods for containing costs in managed care settings have been

   (A) Using gatekeepers
   (B) Physician incentives
   (C) Utilization review
   (D) All of the above

66. Within managed care organizations using gatekeepers, which group is usually designated to be the gatekeepers?

   (A) Primary care physicians
   (B) Clinic administrators
   (C) Specialists
   (D) Chart reviewers

67. Managed care track record of success includes which of the following?

   (A) Reduced hospital admissions
   (B) Containment of health care costs
   (C) Reduction of laboratory tests and procedures
   (D) Reduced referrals to specialists
   (E) All of the above

68. Negative effects of higher penetration of managed care include

   (A) Reduced continuity of care
   (B) Impaired patient-physician communication
   (C) Reduced emphasis on research, teaching, and training
   (D) Shifting of primary patient responsibility from the doctor to the plan
   (E) All of the above

69. A large health maintenance organization (HMO) with computerized medical records did a retrospective study of the type of drug treatment and incidence of myocardial infarction over 4 years in their patients. The study examined whether patients given calcium channel blockers experienced a different rate of myocardial infarction (MI) compared to those given beta blockers. The results showed a rate of MI of 10 in 1000 in the standard therapy versus 16 in 1000 with calcium blockers, $P = 0.03$. What kind of study design did the HMO likely use?

   (A) Clinical trial
   (B) Crossover study
   (C) Case-control study
   (D) Health services research study
   (E) All of the above

70. What are the possible interpretations of this study result?

   (A) Calcium blockers are causing myocardial infarction
   (B) Diuretics and beta blockers are preventing myocardial infarctions
   (C) Physicians are more likely to render treatment to patients at higher risk for myocardial infarction with calcium blockers rather than diuretics
   (D) Treatment selection bias is likely operating
   (E) All of the above

71. Case-control studies contribute most to scientific investigation by

(A) raising important clinical questions (hypotheses), which can then be examined using a clinical trial

(B) comparing the results for consistency with other case-controlled studies on the same topic to look for consistency

(C) providing data to add to other similar case-control studies pooling using meta-analysis to establish causation

(D) providing a quick and relatively inexpensive method for answering important clinical treatment questions

72. What is the most serious problem with analyzing clinic observational data to look for benefits of treatment? For example, an observational study result finding that heart failure patients treated with ACE inhibitors have a higher mortality rate compared with patients receiving no drug treatment.

(A) Incomplete data in clinical records

(B) Treatment selection bias

(C) Misdiagnosis of heart failure in the clinic

(D) Loss to follow-up

73. An aggressive state vaccination program results in 90% of high school aged children vaccinated against measles. Even with 10% of children not vaccinated, the state has only a trivial number of cases of measles reported. Why was the vaccination program so successful?

(A) Some children were vaccinated in the past but not aware of it

(B) The vaccine has a very high effectiveness in transferring immunity

(C) Many cases of measles went unreported

(D) The phenomenon of herd immunity

74. Which of the following is an example of passive immunity?

(A) Injection of immunoglobulin

(B) Attenuated polio vaccine

(C) Vitamin B injections

(D) None of the above

75. Why have quarantine and isolation been largely discarded as a means to control infectious diseases?

(A) It is too difficult and expensive
(B) Often, carriers are asymptomatic
(C) The policy violates constitutional rights
(D) There is increased risk of infection to health care staff

76. Vaccination is defined as

(A) delivery or administration of a vaccine
(B) the act of immunizing an individual
(C) achieving immunity in a passive way
(D) All of the above

77. Hospitals represent a place where unusual or resistant microorganisms are more likely to occur than in the general community. Why?

(A) There are more immunosuppressed hosts
(B) There is widespread use of antibiotics
(C) There is a higher prevalence of resistant organisms
(D) All of the above

CASE STUDY QUESTIONS

A randomized clinical trial was conducted comparing a promising new antiepileptic drug (miniseize®) to placebo for the treatment of seizures. The study was double blinded and, over the 6-month duration of the study, 60% of patients on the active drug were discontinued from treatment because of side effects; 20% of patients were discontinued from the placebo group. The final results of the study showed a 22% reduction in seizures in the active group and a 19% reduction on placebo. This difference was not statistically significantly different.

78. The most likely explanation of the reduction in seizures in both groups is

(A) placebo effect
(B) regression to the mean
(C) differential rates in study groups off therapy
(D) chance

79. What is the most serious problem with the high rate of active drug group going off treatment?

   (A) Effect on study power
   (B) High dropout rate in the active drug group makes it unethical to continue the trial
   (C) An "on treatment" analysis must be used as the primary analysis
   (D) There is no serious problem

80. The preferred analysis for comparing miniseize® to placebo is to

   (A) analyze the difference in total reported reduction in seizures between groups over the 6 months of follow-up
   (B) examine the difference in seizure incidence between groups after adjustment for dropouts and nonadherence
   (C) use intention to treat analysis
   (D) focus main analysis on special subgroups, for example, men, women, African Americans, whites, or elderly patients.

81. The study physicians realize that the high rate of going off miniseize® will likely bias the results toward a negative result. They reason that only those patients who remained on miniseize® throughout the study could be expected to benefit. To address this problem, an analysis comparing the 40% of patients who took miniseize® regularly to the placebo group patients was done. What was the most likely result in doing this analysis?

   (A) Regular adherers to miniseize® experienced a significant reduction in seizure incidence compared to patients given placebo
   (B) There was no difference from overall analysis (intention to treat)
   (C) The miniseize® group has a higher rate of seizures compared to placebo
   (D) The effect of adherence or endpoint analysis is likely random

82. A manuscript is written on these dramatic results and submitted to a prestigious journal. The journal reviewers send back the paper with a request that an additional analysis be done that compares the adherers to miniseize® to the adherers to placebo. What is the most likely result of this analysis?

 (A) The results are similar to the original analysis, showing a marked reduction in seizures with miniseize® in active drug adherers versus the whole placebo group
 (B) The results of this analysis are random and not predictable
 (C) The analysis recommended by the journal reviewers is not required because a highly statistically significant effect has been shown with miniseize®
 (D) The seizure rate in the miniseize® adherers is lower than the overall rate (8%), but so is the seizure rate in the placebo adherers (9%), and this comparison is not statistically significant

83. Assuming that the result of this analysis of adherers shows an equally low rate of seizures in the adherers of both miniseize® and placebo and that this comparison was not statistically significant, what is a reasonable explanation of this result?

 (A) Type II error
 (B) Caios theory
 (C) Statistics "lie"
 (D) Adherers are different from nonadherers in ways not related to the drugs they are taking (e.g., they are more health conscious)

84. Which of the following is one of the main lessons to the investigators of this study?

 (A) Subgrouping after randomization based on response (responders versus nonresponders) should not be done
 (B) Clinical judgment is more reliable than statistically manipulated study results
 (C) The study design evaluation of miniseize® is flawed
 (D) A study with more statistical power would not have had these problems

85. In the Joint National Committee VI report, which nonpharmacologic method is strongly recommended for the treatment and prevention of high blood pressure?

    (A) Meditation
    (B) Dietary sodium reduction
    (C) Weight loss
    (D) Increased physical activity
    (E) All of the above

86. Physicians who measure blood pressure are more likely to prefer which terminal digit?

    (A) Two
    (B) Four
    (C) Zero
    (D) Six
    (E) Eight

87. The science of biostatistics is essentially a study of

    (A) means
    (B) modes
    (C) mortality trends
    (D) variability in biologic measures

88. Unresolved issues between managed care and practicing physicians include

    (A) reimbursement rates for medical services
    (B) quality of care
    (C) cost of care
    (D) malpractice liability
    (E) all of the above

89. One of the main differences between a staff model health maintenance organization (HMO) and a preferred provider organization (PPO) is that

    (A) HMOs put more emphasis on disease prevention
    (B) in a staff model, HMO physicians are salaried, and in a PPO, physicians are reimbursed at contractual rates
    (C) PPOs have broader coverage in outpatient services
    (D) PPOs are primarily hospital-centered care

90. What is the test statistic used with analysis of variance (ANOVA)?

(A) F statistic
(B) Z statistic
(C) Chi square
(D) Bonferonni

91. A clinical trial was carried out comparing a new nonsteroidal antiinflammatory agent to placebo for osteoarthritic joint pain. The reduction in reported pain episodes was reduced with the drug by 25% compared to placebo. This study was a small pilot study; however, the P value of the t-test was 0.20. What does this value indicate?

(A) This outcome would be expected by chance in 10 of 20 similar studies
(B) This result is not clinically meaningful
(C) This outcome occurred by chance
(D) This specific result would have been expected in one of five studies carried out with this study design

92. What is a potential explanation for the results in question 91?

(A) Type I error was made
(B) Inappropriate study design for this question
(C) Type II error was made
(D) Study groups were too diverse

93. What could be done to address the study's problems identified in question 92?

(A) Increase the sample size
(B) Extend follow-up and increase the events
(C) Enhance drug adherence in both groups
(D) All of the above

94. What type of accident accounts for up to 50% of all accidental deaths in the United States?

(A) Gun accidents
(B) Occupational accidents
(C) Poisoning accidents
(D) Motor vehicle accidents

95. Worldwide, what is the most common means of transmission of human immunodeficiency virus?

(A) Male homosexual contact
(B) Casual contact
(C) Intravenous drug use
(D) Heterosexual contact
(E) Blood products

96. What means of transmission of human immunodeficiency virus has decreased substantially?

(A) Male homosexual contact
(B) Infusion of blood and blood products
(C) Intravenous drug use
(D) None of the above

97. Which of the following areas worldwide have extraordinarily high rates of infection with human immunodeficiency virus?

(A) Southeast Asia
(B) Indian subcontinent
(C) Sub-Saharan Africa
(D) All of the above

98. Which of the following screening tests for newborns is mandatory in most states?

(A) Neural tube defects
(B) Phenylketonuria
(C) Ventricular septal defects
(D) Hyperthyroidism

99. In addition to phenylketonuria, what other condition is recommended for widespread screening in newborns?

(A) Wilms' tumor
(B) Diabetes mellitus
(C) Congential hypothyroidism
(D) Tay-Sachs disease

100. What is the most desirable method for filling out death certificates?

   (A) Recording only the primary underlying cause of death
   (B) Recording the primary cause of death and comorbid conditions
   (C) Recording the primary cause of death and other causes
   (D) None of the above

101. The process of death certification in the United States works best for

   (A) tracking changes in disease incidence over time
   (B) ensuring a high autopsy percentage of deaths
   (C) determining the diagnostic validity of the death certificate
   (D) all of the above

102. In the United States, although men generally have a higher death rate than women, for which of the following conditions are death rates similar in both genders?

   (A) Diabetes mellitus
   (B) Solid tumor cancers
   (C) Chronic lung disease
   (D) Accidents and suicide

103. Infant mortality rates are frequently used as a measure of the effectiveness of public health programs. What are the limitations in using infant mortality rate figures?

   (A) Infant mortality rates do not account for chronic diseases
   (B) Infant mortality rates exaggerate the effectiveness of environmental health and communicable diseases
   (C) Mortality rates in older individuals are not accounted for
   (D) Infant mortality rates do not account for the effects of mental illness
   (E) All of the above

104. An "intention to treat" analysis is defined as

   (A) analysis for which only patients undergoing treatment are included
   (B) analysis in which nonadherers to drug are excluded from the analysis
   (C) analysis of only those patients on treatment at the end of the trial
   (D) inclusion of all patients randomized into the study, whether or not they remained on the study drug during the trial

105. What is the main reason for the increase in recent years of drug-resistant organisms?

   (A) Lack of antiviral drugs
   (B) Overuse of antibiotics
   (C) Poor patient compliance
   (D) Development of new antibiotic drugs

106. Which communicable disease has been completely eradicated through aggressive vaccination programs?

   (A) Herpes virus
   (B) Measles
   (C) Poliomyelitis
   (D) Smallpox

107. The illustration shows a plot of a small observation study frequency distribution. There are 18 patients. The mean systolic blood pressure of the group is 124 mmHg. The median in this set of measurements is

   (A) 124 mmHg
   (B) 122 mmHg
   (C) 130 mmHg
   (D) 123 mmHg

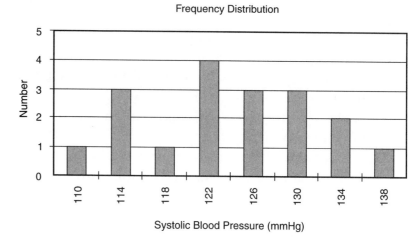

Frequency distribution.

108. The mode in this data set is

(A) 126 mmHg
(B) 123 mmHg
(C) 122 mmHg
(D) 130 mmHg

109. In health services research an "efficacy" study is best described as

(A) A clinical trial
(B) Assessing benefit of a treatment under ideal conditions
(C) An outcome study
(D) A case-control study

110. Outcomes research has traditionally used which type of study design?

(A) Effectiveness
(B) Cost-benefit
(C) Efficacy
(D) Observational

111. A study examining the effect of nicotine patches to aid patients in quitting smoking carried out in a typical community setting is

(A) an effectiveness study
(B) a cost-effectiveness study
(C) an efficacy study
(D) an observational study
(E) none of the above

112. Health services research includes which method of investigation?

(A) Quality
(B) Costs
(C) Organization of services
(D) Outcomes
(E) All of the above

113. It was noticed in the 1950s from the Framingham Heart Study data and from other studies that a subfraction of serum cholesterol (α) or HDL-C was inversely related to risk of cardiovascular disease (CVD). Total cholesterol was noted to be strongly and positively related to risk of CVD. It took more than 2 decades before HDL-C was accepted as a bona fide risk factor. Why?

(A) The association was weak
(B) HDL-C was not related in graded fashion to CVD
(C) The temporal relation was reversed
(D) There was no biologic probability

114. Which of the following methods of infection control are largely ineffective in the community?

(A) Isolation and quarantine
(B) Improved nutrition and hygiene
(C) Antibiotics
(D) None of the above

115. In genetic screening prenatally, an elevated serum alpha-fetoprotein (AFP) is associated with what defect?

(A) Down syndrome
(B) Neural tube defect
(C) Cleft palate
(D) Hyperbilirubinemia

116. In most US states, what abnormality is routinely screened for in newborns?

(A) Phenylketonuria
(B) Congenital hypothyroidism
(C) Hemoglobinopathies
(D) Galactosemia
(E) All of the above

117. What prenatal screening method is used the earliest (at 10 to 11 weeks' gestation)?

(A) Maternal plasma
(B) Amniocentesis
(C) Fetal plasma
(D) Chorionic villus sampling

118. Of what percentage of the more than 65,000 commercial chemicals are the health hazards known?

(A) 40%
(B) 10%
(C) 33%
(D) 2%

119. The American Red Cross carried out a community blood cholesterol screening program. People with levels above 250 mg/dl were referred to their personal doctor for evaluation. Of the 98 people referred, 80 visited their own physicians for retesting. On retesting, only 45 of the 80 still had serum cholesterol as high as 250 mg/dl. What is the most likely explanation of the smaller prevalence of abnormal values on retest?

(A) Patients were not fasting at the initial screening
(B) Regression to the mean
(C) Laboratory error
(D) Patients changed their diet between the two cholesterol measures

120. Analysis of a clinic's blood pressure measurements found that 60% of the systolic and diastolic values ended in the terminal digit "0." Only 8% ended in "2." What most likely explains this difference?

(A) Staff is not trained to obtain blood pressures
(B) Inappropriate staff members are allowed to do measurements
(C) The equipment is not functioning correctly
(D) There is observer bias

121. The group of "physician extenders" currently being trained and studied in the United States includes such personnel as

(A) nurse practitioners
(B) licensed practical nurses
(C) occupational therapists
(D) physical therapy assistants
(E) all of the above

122. A questionnaire mailed to 1000 adult women asked about the presence or absence of joint stiffness. Of these women, 500 returned the questionnaire, and 100 stated that they had stiff joints. The appropriate rate for the prevalence of stiff joints would be

(A) 100 in 1000, if the questionnaires are correctly answered
(B) 100 in 500, if the nonrespondents are similar to the respondents
(C) 500 in 1000, if women with stiff joints are likely not to reply
(D) none of the above

123. Cancer of the colon is more likely to develop in Japanese migrants to Hawaii than Japanese who live in Japan. This difference is best explained by which of the following?

(A) Migrants from a country may differ from those remaining in the country
(B) Hawaii may have environmental carcinogens that are absent in Japan
(C) Japanese living in Hawaii may eat different foods from those eaten by Japanese living in Japan
(D) All of the above factors may contribute

124. In recent decades, the US public has come to believe that health care is a human right. The response of government to this demand has been mainly at the federal level, primarily because

(A) State and local governments have no authority to respond

(B) Many state governors disagree with the "human right" view

(C) Local government officials have neither the training nor the experience to respond

(D) Federal government officials are more sensitive to public demands

(E) Financial resources are most abundant at the federal level

125. When a measurement, such as blood pressure level, leads to a diagnosis of disease or no disease, the cutoff point between the two groups may be defined by

(A) statistical means, such as two standard deviations from the age-specific average

(B) clinical means, such as the level at which symptoms and complications become more frequent

(C) prognosis, such as an elevated risk of future disease

(D) any of the above means, depending on the purpose of the cutoff point

126. A small study attempted to guide health planners as to whether death certificates for esophageal cancer form a useful guide to the frequency of that disease. Its findings were (1) 74 diagnosed before death, (2) 53 confirmed at autopsy, (3) 21 not confirmed at autopsy, and (4) 22 first diagnosed at autopsy. Indicate which of the following statements is correct.

(A) 22 of 74 of individual cases were missed before death

(B) The false-positive diagnoses before death approximately balance the false-negative diagnoses

(C) Autopsies are essential to obtain the approximate population frequency

(D) All of the above

127. The average expectation of life at birth

(A) increases with improvements in health
(B) decreases as death rates increase
(C) is higher for US females than males
(D) has all of the above characteristics

128. The legal requirement that physicians report selected diseases

(A) has succeeded particularly for mental illnesses
(B) gives an incomplete picture of disease incidence
(C) has been used mainly for noninfectious conditions
(D) has slowed the control of infectious disease

129. Epidemiologic studies of disease usually involve

(A) both people with and without the disease under study
(B) discarding the clinical knowledge of disease
(C) emphasizing the cases of advanced disease
(D) relating local cases to the national population

130. The frequency of much infectious disease can best be explained by

(A) host factors
(B) characteristics of the infectious agent
(C) environmental factors
(D) interaction of all of the above

131. A clinical trial is "double blind" when

(A) the subjects know that they belong to the control group
(B) the investigators do not fully understand the pathology of the condition
(C) neither the physician (investigator) nor patient knows the study group assignment
(D) all of the above conditions are met

132. In an epidemic of food poisoning, the contaminated food must

    (A) be eaten by patients in all cases
    (B) have been avoided by all who remained well
    (C) be consumed by patients in most of the cases and by only a few of the well (non-cases)
    (D) be characterized by none of the above

133. In the United States, the Public Health Service is

    (A) a federal agency with many public health functions
    (B) the agency using about two thirds of the federal health budget
    (C) the guide for the activities of PROs
    (D) the federal agency responsible for Medicare and Medicaid
    (E) all of the above

134. The prevention and better control of hypertension involve

    (A) obesity control, reduced salt and alcohol intake, and increased physical activity
    (B) long-term antihypertensive treatment in established cases
    (C) more extensive screening for elevated blood pressure in employees
    (D) all of the above

135. Which of the following can adversely influence pregnancy and infant health?

    (A) Smoking
    (B) Alcohol use
    (C) Untreated diabetes
    (D) All of the above

136. The delivery of routine immunizations could be widened by

    (A) eliminating charges for these procedures
    (B) funding preventive measures through government subsidies
    (C) offering vaccines free to physicians who do not charge their patients for immunizations
    (D) all of the above measures

137. Identifying the environmental causes of disease is complicated because

    (A) the period may be short between exposure and disease onset
    (B) clear data that reveal the actual associations are usually available but are overlooked
    (C) many agents may contribute to the same disease
    (D) all of the above reasons play a part

138. The Health Care Financing Administration is a

    (A) voluntary agency that funds health care
    (B) philanthropic association, such as the Rockefeller Foundation
    (C) professional association that funds health administrators
    (D) federal agency within the PHS responsible for Medicare and Medicaid

139. Randomization into a clinical trial is best characterized by which of the following?

    (A) Group assignment is unknown to the participant
    (B) There is an equal chance of group assignment
    (C) Group assignment is unpredictable
    (D) Group assignment is sequential

140. Which of the following best describes the "population perspective" on disease prevention in the community?

    (A) To most efficiently prevent disease, only high-risk individuals (e.g., patients with hyperlipidemia, hypertensive patients) should receive treatment
    (B) Lowering risk factors by a substantial amount in high-risk patients and patients with clinical disease will achieve the best results in preventing the disease
    (C) Lowering the population mean level of the risk factor (e.g., blood cholesterol levels, blood pressure) by only a small percent will shift the entire population distribution of the risk factor and prevent the most disease
    (D) It is not possible for populations to change their risk levels significantly

141. What is the "gold standard" in research for evaluating the efficacy of new therapies?

    (A) Case-control study
    (B) Case history
    (C) A prospective observational study
    (D) Clinical trial

142. Case-control studies are useful for

    (A) studying diseases that are rare
    (B) generating causal hypotheses
    (C) estimating risk for an exposure
    (D) all of the above

143. Which of the following is the most efficient and least costly method of establishing benefit of a treatment?

    (A) Prospective clinical trial
    (B) Case-control study
    (C) Prospective observational study
    (D) Meta-analysis—pooling results of several clinical trials

144. Which of the following is not one of the seven epidemiologic criteria used for inferring causation?

    (A) sensitivity
    (B) independence
    (C) specificity
    (D) temporality

145. What term is used to describe the ratio of true-positive tests to all tests that are positive (true-positives plus false-positives)?

    (A) Sensitivity
    (B) Positive predictive value
    (C) Specificity
    (D) Congruence

146. Which of the following statements in a clinical trial evaluating a new treatment's effect best describes the meaning of the term "$P < 0.05$"?

   (A) The outcome is statistically significant and therefore clinically important
   (B) A type II, or beta, error has likely occurred
   (C) One must reject the alternative hypothesis
   (D) If a similar experiment was carried out repeatedly, one would expect the observed result to occur less than 5% of the time by chance, given the variability of measures in the study

147. The statistical power of a study is related to

   (A) the type II, or beta, error
   (B) the treatment difference from control
   (C) sample size
   (D) all of the above

148. In a study, hypertensive patients with diastolic blood pressures of more than 95 mmHg were selected as subjects. These patients were randomized to two new dietary treatments: (1) potassium supplementation and (2) calcium supplementation. Baseline diastolic blood pressure was 102 mmHg. After 6 weeks, diastolic blood pressure changed by -12 ± 5 (standard error of difference) in the potassium group and by -11 ± 4 in the calcium group. What is the most likely explanation for the favorable reduction in blood pressure?

   (A) Potassium and calcium both are equally effective in lowering blood pressure
   (B) Neither is effective. Regression to the mean can explain the drop in blood pressure
   (C) Placebo effect has occurred
   (D) Errors were made in blood pressure measurement

149. What is the most likely explanation for the increased incidence of certain diseases in African Americans versus whites?

   (A) Race-related genetic differences
   (B) Inherent susceptibility of races to different diseases
   (C) Differences in access to health care
   (D) Environmental and socioeconomic differences

150. In 1992, what disease in many US cities was the most common cause of death in men aged 25 to 44 years?

(A) AIDS
(B) Cancer
(C) Hypertensive stroke
(D) Drug overdose

151. Which cardiovascular risk factor has not decreased in age-adjusted incidence over the last decade?

(A) Systolic blood pressure
(B) Serum cholesterol
(C) Cigarette smoking
(D) Obesity

152. In the United States, compared to whites, African Americans have an increased adjusted mortality and morbidity rate for which of the following?

(A) Coronary heart disease
(B) Lung cancer
(C) Diabetes
(D) Cancer
(E) Virtually all diseases

153. Which of the following statements is not correct?

(A) Racial classifications are based on genetic biologic differences
(B) Race is intertwined closely with socioeconomic conditions
(C) Race is related to risk of developing the disease for many conditions
(D) The most likely explanation for racial differences in disease is environment, not genetics

154. Which type of cancer risk is not associated with cigarette smoking?

(A) Bladder
(B) Larynx
(C) Colon
(D) Pancreas
(E) Lung

155. Which of the following is the single most preventable cause of death in the United States?

(A) Alcohol
(B) Chemical carcinogens
(C) Physical inactivity
(D) Cigarette smoking

156. Which of the following best describes the concept of statistical power?

(A) The chance of falsely assuming a treatment effect
(B) Depends solely on the sample size of the study
(C) The likelihood that there is no type II error
(D) The overall clinical significance of the study results

157. Regression to the mean can be minimized or essentially eliminated by use of

(A) averaging multiple measures
(B) standardizing measurement procedures
(C) using a baseline value for which exclusion criteria were not applied
(D) all of the above

158. Which blood pressure measurement most strongly relates to risk of developing cardiovascular disease?

(A) Systolic blood pressure
(B) Diastolic blood pressure
(C) Mean blood pressure
(D) Ambulatory blood pressure

159. Lowering systolic blood pressure in adults 60 years of age and older with isolated systolic hypertension (systolic blood pressure greater than or equal to 160 mmHg and diastolic blood pressure less than or equal to 90 mmHg) will significantly reduce

(A) cardiovascular disease
(B) fatal and nonfatal combined stroke
(C) congestive heart failure
(D) all of the above

160. Approximately what percent of the United States adult population smoked cigarettes in 1999?

(A) 23%
(B) 15%
(C) 33%
(D) 40%
(E) none of the above

161. By what means does the United States federal government encourage states to set age 21 as the legal minimal age to drink alcohol?

(A) Information and education directed at state health departments
(B) Providing block grants
(C) Political lobbying
(D) Restricting a portion of highway construction funds

162. What is currently the most prevalent treatment approach for chemical dependency?

(A) Behavioral modification techniques
(B) Twelve-step programs
(C) Aversive conditioning
(D) Medication (e.g., disulfiram, sedatives)

163. Compared to higher income groups, lower income groups have

(A) higher infant mortality rates
(B) higher rates of acquiring most infectious disease
(C) higher prevalence of hypertension
(D) higher rate of dental disease
(E) all of the above

164. In recent years, what factors are not responsible for the increased costs of health care?

(A) Increased wages for health care personnel
(B) New medical technology
(C) Increased levels of hospital productivity
(D) Training of physicians and nurses

165. What system, legislated in the United States in 1982 and based on diagnostic codes, concerns detailed payments for Medicare hospital inpatients?

(A) DRGs
(B) HMOs
(C) PPOs
(D) OSHA
(E) EPA

1-B Lifestyle changes in the population such as weight loss and sodium reduction can potentially be very effective in preventing disease (e.g., cardiovascular disease) from the population perspective. That is, small changes, such as 2 to 3 mmHg in systolic blood pressure, can shift the entire distribution of the population and therefore substantially prevent disease. In this case, most cardiovascular disease occurs in the population of people who have average or above average risk factors. High-risk patients experience even higher rates of disease, but there are few high-risk patients in the population compared to average or above average patients. The latter group makes up the majority of cardiovascular disease cases that occur in the community.

2-D See answer to question 1.

3-B The total amount of heart disease prevention would occur at the above average to high normal levels because there are so many people in these groups. However, the absolute risk in the individual is higher in the high-risk group.

4-C Funeral director.

5-D The attending physician.

6-B A nosologist is a specialist who interprets the attending physician's data and assigns the final cause of death.

7-E All of the above. Crude death rate is influenced by differences in the population being studied.

8-A Although obesity in the United States is highly prevalent in all race and gender subgroups, African Americans have the highest prevalence of obesity (48.6%) followed by Hispanic women (46.7%) and Hispanic men (35.5%). White women and white men have the lowest prevalence at (32.9%) and (32.3%), respectively.

9-D The average increase in weight is 8 pounds. This is an alarming increase especially when considering the relatively short time frame.

10-C Lack of and reduced physical activity is thought to be the most important contributor to the increased rates of obesity.

11-A 99.7%.

12-B Normal distributions are frequently referred to as Gaussian.

13-B According to the more conservative National Institutes of Health guidelines on the number of Americans who are obese, the number is approximately 100 million (body mass index greater than or equal to 30). The NHANES III estimate was 58 million.

14-D Although waist-to-hip ratio was the most common measure of central obesity, waist circumference is as reliable or more so and is much easier to perform with less variation.

15-D Body mass index (BMI) is the preferred measure. BMI is weight in kilograms divided by height in centimeters squared (weight/height^2).

16-C According to NIH guidelines, patients should be assessed for obesity every 2 years.

17-C High risk is defined as a body mass index (BMI) greater than or equal to 30 regardless of risk factors, or BMI greater than or equal to 27 with at least two risk factors needed before considering drug therapy.

18-E Diabetes, high blood pressure, high cholesterol levels, and sleep apnea are all risk factors for consideration in drug treatment of obesity.

19-A Observed associations in case-control studies cannot establish causation. Case-control study results frequently raise important questions but cannot definitively answer the question. Case-control studies are much less costly than clinical trials but are not as good for evaluating medical treatments. Case-control studies are more subject to treatment selection bias.

20-E Defining the endpoint, standardization of measure, similar contact frequency, and blinded observers doing the ascertainment are all useful in eliminating or reducing endpoint ascertainment bias.

21-D The study with only 15 patients per group lacks statistical power and most likely made a type II error. A type I error would have been a false-positive result. A two-group, parallel, randomized trial is an excellent design for this question; however, the sample size would need to be much larger for the treatment difference observed.

22-B Power relates to when a false-negative assumption is made or the probability of not making a type II error. Power is mainly a concern when study results show no significant difference.

23-A Although all the answers may play a role, the most likely explanation is that treatment selection bias is working. Because diuretics are a treatment for CHF, their use could likely be a surrogate for disease severity.

24-D Double-blind is when the investigator and the patient are blinded to their treatments. The main benefit is to reduce observer measurement bias. Reduced endpoint ascertainment bias is usually done by having the endpoints processed by outside experts wherein the study group designation is also blinded. Credibility is a factor in choosing to blind a study, but it is not the main factor.

25-B Regression to the mean. If the baseline measure utilized a cutpoint different from the mean to enter study subjects, then their patients were caught at that point on the high side of their individual variability (their own BP pattern of variation) of the factor. The next group of measures performed will move or regress to the mean. For example, if the study cutpoint for entering hypertensive patients into a study was greater than or equal to 95 mmHg and mean of the population was 80 mmHg, then the greater than or equal to 95 mmHg group will, on the next clinic visit, have average blood pressures closer to the mean, 92 mmHg.

26-C All statin drugs can potentially reduce LDL-C by 20% to 40% in most patients with high LDL-C levels.

27-A It is estimated from meta-analysis of multiple trial data from LDL-C lowering studies that, for a 1% reduction in LDL-C, there is on average a 2% to 3% reduction in CHD risk.

28-A Cigarette smoking is the single most identifiable cause of death in the United States and one of the largest worldwide. Although diabetes mellitus (juvenile and adult onset) is associated with extremely high risk, diabetes is not as common and is mainly a risk factor for vascular disease. Smoking is a major risk factor for vascular disease and many other diseases such as cancer, chronic lung disease, and infections.

29-A In 1987, lung cancer surpassed breast cancer as the most common cause of death attributed to cancer in women. This increase has been largely attributed to the increasing number of women who started smoking cigarettes in the 1940s, 1950s, and 1960s.

30-D The Multiple Risk Factor Intervention Trial found within 1 year of quitting smoking, there was approximately a 50% reduction in myocardial infarction in the special intervention group compared to usual care.

31-B Although physician advice, history of quit attempts, and spousal support are all positive and useful in quitting smoking, the most powerful prediction of quitting smoking is the number of cigarettes smoked daily. Light smokers are more than twice as likely to quit compared to heavy smokers.

32-A Twenty-five percent of all deaths in the United States are attributed to cigarette smoking. Other major CHD risk factors are increased blood pressure, elevated blood lipid levels, and diabetes mellitus.

33-A Although in general the incidence of smoking has increased in all subgroups of adolescents, African-American teenagers have the highest level of increased incidence.

34-A The National Health and Nutrition Examination Study (NHANES II, Phase 2) was the most recent and was conducted in 1991 to 1994. NHANES II, phase 1, was carried out in 1988 to 1991, and NHANES I in 1975 to 1979.

35-D The Centers for Disease Control and Prevention (CDC) publishes the *Mortality and Morbidity Weekly Report* (MMWR). This is on the required reading list for responsible practicing physicians.

36-A Although obesity is more common in women, it is epidemic in both genders. African-American women have the highest prevalence of obesity of the ethnicity/gender subgroups at 48.6%.

37-D All the options are reasonable hypotheses derived from case-control studies. A controlled clinical trial would need to be carried out to answer the question—Does estrogen replacement prevent coronary heart disease?

38-D All of the above.

39-B A large clinical trial with sufficient power to ensure a low probability of type II error is the standard for gauging causation and effect of treatment. Meta-analysis is limited by publication bias. Journal reviews and clinical judgment are often wrong compared to treatments tested using clinical trials.

40-D All of the above. Study dropouts are likely to be different from active participants in a number of ways.

41-E Since the mid-1970s, obesity has increased in patients of all ages, races, and genders.

42-A Case-control studies can show strength of association but do not establish causation. For example, calcium channel blockers may cause CHD; but, another explanation is that doctors are more likely to use calcium blockers in patients susceptible to CHD.

43-A Toxemia of pregnancy.

44-D Type II errors are also referred to as beta (β) errors, and type I errors are also alpha (α) errors. A type II error relates to the result of no effect and how confident the investigators are that the result truly is no effect.

45-C Control of childhood infectious diseases through better sanitation, immunization, and antibiotics is the primary reason that life expectancy has increased dramatically since the early 1900s.

46-A The Joint National Committee. This group of experts is convened approximately every 4 years by the National High Blood Pressure Education Program of the National Heart, Lung and Blood Institute.

47-C NHANES III results show that only 27% of hypertensive patients in the United States had their disease under control (less than 140/less than 90 mmHg) in the mid-1990s. This figure is down from 29% in the late-1980s.

48-C Leveled off, in part, because there has been no further improvement in blood pressure control.

49-C In the mid-1990s, approximately one third of hypertensive patients were still not identified.

50-A Only about half (53%) of hypertensive patients in the United States were treated with drugs in NHANES III (1991 to 1994).

51-B JNC VI recommends that persons in risk group "C," high risk, initially undergo drug treatment combined with lifestyle modifications. Risk group C includes patients with target organ damage (e.g., left ventricular hypertrophy, funduscopic changes, motinuria), clinical cardiovascular disease, or diabetes mellitus. Diabetes is a major CHD risk factor, with risks 3- to 4-fold higher than for nondiabetics.

52-A Results of studies on the effects of relaxation and meditation on blood pressure have been inconsistent. Weight loss, sodium reduction, alcohol reduction, and increased physical activity are the main lifestyle modalities for treating high blood pressure.

53-D Several studies have shown that low-dose diuretic therapy with hydrochlorothiazide and chlorthalidone (12.5 to 25 mg per day) achieves just as much blood pressure lowering and is much less likely to cause metabolic abnormalities (hypokalemia, hyperglycemia, or hyperlipidemia). Clinical trials using low-dose thiazide diuretics have shown them to be very effective in reducing cardiovascular disease mortality and morbidity.

54-E All of these choices are recommended in JNC VI to control high blood pressure.

55-E The Systolic Hypertension Studies in Europe demonstrated the long-acting dihydropyridine calcium blocker Nitrendopine was effective in reducing total stroke (-36%) compared to placebo.

56-C The main public health goal is to prevent the onset of hypertension. The prevention paradigm emphasizes the population perspective.

57-C Any study that has a significant P value by definition has sufficient power. Power is a concern when the result is not statistically significant.

58-D A risk factor is a characteristic that places an individual at higher chance for developing disease.

59-A An independent risk factor is one that cannot be explained by an association with a second factor. Systolic blood pressure, cigarette smoking, and serum cholesterol are all independent risk factors for coronary heart disease.

60-D The most concern regarding study dropouts occurs when the dropout rates are different across study groups. Study dropouts are almost always quite different from participants in potentially important ways, such as adherence to drug regimen, disease endpoints, and smoking. These differences can potentially confound the study results.

61-A Although it would help the study power by increasing the participant recruitment, the best way to approach the differential dropout rate is to put all efforts possible in increasing retention of both groups.

62-C Randomization is the best method to ensure group compatibility. Blocking treatment assignments guarantees the desired number of participants in each study group. Medical evaluations and adjustment of entry criteria will not help.

63-B The main goal of managed care is to provide acceptable quality medical care at reduced costs. Improved communication between patients and physicians, improved quality of care, and prevention of disease are all desirable but they are not the main purpose of managed care.

64-E The challenges for managed care include all the above: quality, cost control, medical education, and prevention.

65-D Cost containment can involve all the above: 1) gatekeepers or going through primary care doctors first, or 2) providing financial incentives for physicians usually designed to decrease utilization and utilization review.

66-A Primary care physicians, mainly family practice and internal medicine physicians, usually serve as gatekeepers.

67-E All of the above.

68-E All of the above.

69-C A case-control study retrospectively compares cases to control subjects. In this case, patients receiving calcium channel blockers are the "cases" and patients receiving the beta blockers are the "controls."

70-E All of the answers are acceptable. Case-control studies are limited in that they cannot separate cause from association.

71-A Case-control studies contribute most to scientific investigation by raising important questions that can then be examined using other investigative methods, such as clinical trials.

72-B Treatment selection bias is a major confounder in observational data. Patients with more severe disease are more likely to undergo treatment and this treatment often serves as a surrogate for disease severity.

73-D Herd immunity is the phenomenon in which community protection is accomplished at only partial levels of immunization.

74-A Immunoglobin shots are an example of passive immunity. Attenuated polio virus is active immunity.

75-B Although all the answers are credible, the primary reason isolation was abandoned is because of the relatively high prevalence of asymptomatic carriers.

76-D All of the above.

77-D All of the answers apply in the hospital setting.

78-B Regression to the mean is most likely the reason; patients with the highest rate of seizures are entered, but on follow-up, both groups tend to migrate in seizure rates toward the mean.

79-A A high rate of patients off drug in a trial dilutes the treatment contrast and therefore minimizes the treatment effect. The smaller the treatment effect, the lower the power of the study.

80-A Because this is a parallel, two-group clinical trial, the best analysis is to examine differences between the groups in the reduction from baseline in number of seizures.

81-A Results of analyses in only those patients who remain on treatment frequently observe different results compared to intention to treat analysis. The result of the former will usually erroneously favor the active treatment group.

82-D Regular adherers to drug and placebo regimens are likely to be quite different from the nonadherers in many ways.

83-D They will overall be more health conscious and lower risk. The on-treatment analysis in which miniseize® adherers were compared to the entire placebo group is ill advised because the assumption of randomization no longer holds.

84-A On-treatment analysis should not be used to answer the primary question. The assumptions of randomization or group comparability are no longer preserved.

85-E All of the above.

86-C Studies have shown that physicians prefer the "0" digit. In fact, 120/80 is the most common pressure recorded by physicians. This is also the level that has conventionally been considered "normal."

87-D Understanding and interpreting biologic variability is the essence of biostatistics.

88-E All of the items listed are important contentious issues between practicing physicians and managed care.

89-B Both staff model health maintenance organizations and preferred provider organizations (PPOs) are forms of managed care. A primary difference is that staff model physicians are usually salaried and PPO physicians are contracted.

90-A F statistic is used in testing analysis of variance; the Z statistic is for student's t-test. Chi square and Bonferonni is a statistical adjustment of significance for testing multiple comparisons.

91-D A *P* value of 0.20 means this result would have occurred by chance 20%, or in one of five similar studies. A *P* value of <0.05 (1 in 20) is conventionally accepted as statistically significant.

92-C One explanation was that a type II error was made; that is, the study was insufficiently powered to answer this question. Another possibility is that there is truly no difference between study groups. Type I errors are a concern only when the study results are positive.

93-D All of the above. Increasing the sample size, increasing the number of events, and improving adherence (increasing treatment effect) would all increase the statistical power.

94-D Motor vehicle accidents are the major cause of deaths from accidents. This is particularly true in younger age groups.

95-D Worldwide, heterosexual contact is the most common means of transmission. In many developing countries, AIDS is endemic and there is a high prevalence of other sexually transmitted diseases.

96-B Transmission by blood and blood products has substantially decreased since blood tests for the human immunodeficiency virus were developed in 1985.

97-D All of the above.

98-B Phenylketonuria.

99-C Congenital hypo thyroidism.

100-B Primary cause and comorbid causes. For example: primary cause—myocardial infarction; contributing comorbidities—congestive heart failure, end-stage renal disease.

101-A Tracking changes in disease incidence over time.

102-A Diabetes mellitus (type II). Diabetes mellitus is a dominant risk factor for cardiovascular disease in women.

103-E All of these are limitations for following changes in disease incidence.

104-D Intention to treat means including all patients randomized in the analysis.

105-B Casual and inappropriate prescription of antibiotics is thought to be the major contributor to the emergence of resistant microorganisms.

106-D Smallpox.

107-A 124 mmHg. The median is the point where equal numbers of data points are on either side.

108-C 122 mmHg is the most common pressure in this data distribution; therefore, it is the mode.

109-B Efficacy studies examine a treatment under ideal conditions. Effectiveness studies evaluate how treatments perform in typical practice settings.

110-A Although all these designs are used in outcomes research, effectiveness has been most commonly used, that is, evaluating the treatment in the actual practice setting.

111-A An effectiveness study is carried out in a typical practice situation. An efficacy study would look at how well the nicotine patch works under ideal clinical trial conditions.

112-E Health services research includes all the methods listed.

113-D All the epidemiologic causal influences except for biologic plausibility were met: strength, response, independence, temporality, specificity, and consistency. In fact, it was counterintuitive that a higher subfraction of cholesterol could be inversely related. Once the transport function of HDL-C was established years later, HDL-C was rapidly adopted as a major cardiovascular disease risk factor.

114-A Early efforts in the preantibiotic age relied heavily on quarantine and isolation. These methods were largely abandoned when it was discovered that many new cases are acquired from asymptomatic carriers.

115-B Neural tube defects. Low alpha-fetoprotein is associated with trisomy 21 (Down syndrome).

116-E All of the above. All states screen for congenital hypothyroidism and phenylketonuria.

117-D Chorionic villus sampling.

118-D 2%, almost none.

119-B Regression to the mean. Fasting has very little effect on serum cholesterol measures. Laboratory differences are a possible partial explanation, but would not account for such a large effect. Diet changes could not account for the large change since they were captured by the screening at the high side of their individual variability. On return, the large majority will be lower; they "regressed to the mean."

120-D Observer bias.

121-A All these groups are considered "physician extenders."

122-B 100 in 500 because the respondents were similar to the non-respondents.

123-D All the factors could potentially explain the difference.

124-E The federal government has more resources.

125-D Because increased risk is determined by blood pressure level, the cutpoint or hypertensive designation is arbitrary; it, therefore, depends on the purpose.

126-D All of the above.

127-D All these factors influence expectation of life at birth.

128-B This requirement is frequently not adhered to and there is a large amount of misreporting.

129-A Epidemiology involves the study of rates of disease. To determine rates, it is essential to know the number of people with and without the disease under study.

130-D All of these are factors in considering the frequency of infectious diseases.

131-C Double-blind (also called masking) is when neither the investigator nor the patient is aware of his or her study group.

132-C The suspect food should be consumed by most of the cases but by only a few of those free of symptoms.

133-E All of the above.

134-D All of these are involved for improving the control of high blood pressure.

135-D All of the above.

136-D All of the above.

137-C Usually many factors contribute significantly to the development of the disease.

138-D HCFA is the federal agency responsible for Medicare and Medicaid.

139-C The essence of randomization is unpredictability. Although patients are usually randomized to an equal number in each group, this is not necessary and studies sometimes use unequal allocation ratios.

140-C The population perspective takes the view of the entire community and states that even minimal shifts in the mean level of the population will result in substantially less (or more if harmful) disease. This is because the largest proportion of the cases will be found within 1 standard deviation from the mean. High-risk patients are at the extremes, but they are far fewer in terms of absolute numbers.

141-D Well-done clinical trials are considered the "gold standard" design for evaluation of the effects of treatments.

142-D All of the above.

143-D Meta-analysis in which the studies are the unit of analysis. This method requires no new data collection.

144-A Although sensitivity is related, it is not one of the seven epidemiologic criteria.

145-B Positive predictive value.

146-D Less than 0.05 means that if the result was positive, one would expect it to occur by chance in less than 5% of similar studies.

147-A All of the above.

148-B Regression to the mean is the observation that when a cutpoint away from the mean is set (e.g., systolic blood pressure greater than or equal to 140) at an initial visit, the individual is more likely to be captured on the high side of his or her within-individual variation of the variable selected. Follow-up measurements are likely to be lower. If the cutpoint set was in fact the mean value, there would be regression to the mean.

149-D Environmental and socioeconomic conditions explain most of the differences in disease frequency among African Americans and whites. To date, genetic differences have only rarely been responsible (e.g., sickle cell anemia). Access to health care also is related to socioeconomic and environmental factors.

150-A AIDS.

151-D Obesity is the only cardiovascular risk factor that has increased in incidence over the past 10 years.

152-E African-Americans have increased risk for almost all diseases (except suicide). This nonspecificity points to socioeconomic and environmental factors as explanations for these differences.

153-A Racial classification is culturally and not biologically determined.

154-C Cigarette smoking has not been found to increase risk for colon cancer.

155-D Cigarette smoking.

156-C Power is the chance of not making a type II error, or the chance of making a false-negative conclusion.

157-D All of the above.

158-A Results of 15 years of follow-up for cause-specific deaths in 362,000 men screened for CHD risk factors between 1973 and 1975 show that systolic pressure is the dominant risk predictor.

159-D All of the above. In the Systolic Hypertension in Elderly Study, total incidence of stroke was reduced by 36%, fatal and nonfatal CHD was reduced by 27%, and heart failure by 54% in a group given low-dose diuretic compared to placebo. Other studies confirmed these results.

160-A 25%.

161-D The threat of restricting highway funding has been a strong incentive for states to have the legal age for alcohol intake set at 21 years.

162-B Although all these techniques have been used, the most widely practiced alcohol intervention involves the 12-step program.

163-E Low income is strongly associated with the chances of developing virtually all diseases.

164-D Physician and nurse training represents a small portion of all health care costs.

165-A DRGs, or diagnosis-related groups.

Community Health
Must-Know Topics

The following must-know topics are discussed in this review. It would be useful for you to formulate outlines of the topics because knowledge of the related material will be key to your understanding of the subject and material and for passing the examination.

- Population perspective

- Vital statistics

- Normal distribution

- Measures of variability

- Statistical testing

- Confounding bias

- Type I, Type II errors/power

- Regression to the mean

- Types of research studies

- Clinical trials

- Meta-analysis

- Epidemiological causation inference

- Sensitivity/specificity

- Managed care

- Ethnicity and health

- High priority health conditions

Index

*Page numbers in *italics* denote figures; those followed by a *t* denote tables.